COPING WITH GOUT

CHRISTINE CRAGGS-HINTON, mother of three, followed a career in the Civil Service until, in 1991, she developed fibromyalgia, a chronic pain condition. Christine took up writing for therapeutic reasons and has, in the past few years, produced *Living with Fibromyalgia*, *The Fibromyalgia Healing Diet*, *The Chronic Fatigue Healing Diet* and *Coping with Polycystic Ovary Syndrome* (all published by Sheldon Press). She also writes for the Fibromyalgia Association UK and the related *FaMily* magazine. In recent years she has become interested in fiction writing, too.

Free form Amino Acid
28g/1oz Cottage Cheese 15 cals
28g/1oz Soya Beans 50 cals
Complex Carbs — recommended
Banana
Orange
apple.
Pasta
Bread
Cabbage.

Overcoming Common Problems Series

Selected titles

A full list of titles is available from Sheldon Press,
36 Causton Street, London SW1P 4ST, and on our website at
www.sheldonpress.co.uk

Assertiveness: Step by Step
Dr Windy Dryden and Daniel Constantinou

Breaking Free
Carolyn Ainscough and Kay Toon

Calm Down
Paul Hauck

Cataract: What You Need to Know
Mark Watts

Cider Vinegar
Margaret Hills

Comfort for Depression
Janet Horwood

Confidence Works
Gladeana McMahon

Coping Successfully with Pain
Neville Shone

Coping Successfully with Panic Attacks
Shirley Trickett

Coping Successfully with Period Problems
Mary-Claire Mason

Coping Successfully with Prostate Cancer
Dr Tom Smith

Coping Successfully with Ulcerative Colitis
Peter Cartwright

Coping Successfully with Your Hiatus Hernia
Dr Tom Smith

Coping Successfully with Your Irritable Bowel
Rosemary Nicol

Coping with Alopecia
Dr Nigel Hunt and Dr Sue McHale

Coping with Anxiety and Depression
Shirley Trickett

Coping with Blushing
Dr Robert Edelmann

Coping with Bowel Cancer
Dr Tom Smith

Coping with Brain Injury
Maggie Rich

Coping with Candida
Shirley Trickett

Coping with Chemotherapy
Dr Terry Priestman

Coping with Childhood Allergies
Jill Eckersley

Coping with Childhood Asthma
Jill Eckersley

Coping with Chronic Fatigue
Trudie Chalder

Coping with Coeliac Disease
Karen Brody

Coping with Cystitis
Caroline Clayton

Coping with Depression and Elation
Patrick McKeon

Coping with Down's Syndrome
Fiona Marshall

Coping with Dyspraxia
Jill Eckersley

Coping with Eating Disorders and Body Image
Christine Craggs-Hinton

Coping with Eczema
Dr Robert Youngson

Coping with Endometriosis
Jo Mears

Coping with Epilepsy
Fiona Marshall and
Dr Pamela Crawford

Coping with Fibroids
Mary-Claire Mason

Coping with Gout
Christine Craggs-Hinton

Coping with Heartburn and Reflux
Dr Tom Smith

Coping with Incontinence
Dr Joan Gomez

Coping with Long-Term Illness
Barbara Baker

Coping with Macular Degeneration
Dr Patricia Gilbert

Coping with the Menopause
Janet Horwood

Overcoming Common Problems Series

Overcoming Common Problems Series

Overcoming Common Problems

Coping with Gout

Christine Craggs-Hinton

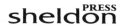

First published in Great Britain in 2004

Sheldon Press
36 Causton Street
London SW1P 4ST

British Library Cataloguing-in-Publication Data

A catalogue record for this book is available from the British Library

ISBN-13: 978–0–85969–922–8
ISBN-10: 0–85969–922–6

3 5 7 9 10 8 6 4 2

Typeset by Deltatype Limited, Birkenhead, Merseyside
Printed by Ashford Colour Press

Contents

Acknowledgements

I would like to say a special thank you to:

David Craggs-Hinton, my husband, not only for his love and support, but also for being the eternal fount of wisdom and knowledge from which I ceaselessly draw.

Walter Hinton, my father-in-law, for his many insights into life with gout and for being the kindest man who would do anything for his family.

Introduction

For centuries, gout was known as 'the disease of kings and plenty' – the result of overindulgence in food and drink. Indeed, in the seventeenth to nineteenth centuries much fun was poked at the condition by lampoonists, who delighted in ridiculing the wealthier classes. Unfortunately, old notions have lingered on, and even now individuals can face laughter when they reveal their diagnosis. However, this condition can be exceedingly painful, as anyone who suffers from it will confirm. It certainly doesn't warrant merriment.

In the past, the reasoning that gout was a disease of excess influenced the lack of significant medical progress into its causes and treatment, despite its having been observed for two thousand years. It is only in the last hundred years that great advances have been made. Indeed, research into gout represents a victory for medical investigation. We now have the ability to correct the condition in some patients and to treat it effectively in others. There is no magic potion, however. Coping successfully with gout depends largely on the sufferer working closely with their doctor and being committed to certain diet and lifestyle changes. The necessary changes are described in this book, along with information about medications, complementary therapies and emotional help.

> People wish their enemies dead – but I do not.
> I say give them the gout, give them the stone!
> > (Lady Mary Wortley Montagu,
> > in a letter to Horace Walpole.)

1

What is Gout?

Gout is a form of acute arthritis that usually affects the joints. However, it may also present itself in one or more of the tendons, in the cartilage or as lumps (known as tophi) under the skin.

The condition is characterized by the following symptoms:

- tenderness and pain (often severe)
- inflammation
- swelling
- reddening
- a mild fever

An attack of acute gout – sometimes called acute gouty arthritis – will normally come on suddenly and swiftly, generally overnight. The affected area will start to feel hot and the skin will become red and appear shiny. Within an hour or so, it may become so painful that even the bedclothes start to feel too heavy. In many cases the individual may also develop a mild fever. The term gout is derived from the Latin word *gutta*, which means a drop – probably because it felt like red hot liquid dropping on to the area concerned. Gout is recognized as being one of the most painful conditions in medicine.

Although gout is usually associated with the base of the big toe, any joint in the body can be affected, and occasionally it can strike at more than one joint at once. Other areas affected can be the heel, ankle, knee, hand, wrist or elbow. However, it is thought that over half of first attacks affect the big toe. The patient will often limp into the doctor's surgery wearing an open-toed sandal, as contact with shoes or socks can intensify the pain.

If left untreated a mild attack may last for a few days, but a severe attack can persist for several weeks, with some residual pain and discomfort for a further few weeks. After the attack, the area typically returns to normal. However, once the individual has experienced an initial attack, the chances are that other attacks will follow, becoming more painful each time and affecting further areas. In time, the pain will not resolve itself between flare-ups and disability ensues. Fortunately, with diet and lifestyle adjustments – and with medications should you wish to go down that route – the progress of the disease can be halted.

Who gets gout?

Gout occurs in adults of both sexes, but is thought to be at least ten times more common in men than in women. Levels of a chemical called uric acid (urate) tend to increase in men at puberty, and because it takes at least 20 years of raised levels to cause the symptoms of gout, men commonly develop it in their late thirties and through their forties. Women typically develop gout in later life, often in their sixties and seventies. According to some experts, oestrogen – the 'female' hormone – protects against raised levels of uric acid, and when oestrogen levels fall during menopause, levels of uric acid begin to build up.

A recent survey by market analysts Taylor Nelson Sofres found that three per cent of adults questioned had experienced gout.

What causes gout?

Gout is usually linked to raised levels of uric acid (urate) in the blood. Everyone has some uric acid. However, it is generally harmless and eliminated with the urine. It is only when levels are higher than normal that problems can occur.

What is uric acid (urate)?

Uric acid is a type of metabolic waste that cannot be broken down within the body. It is formed in the liver as the body degrades other waste products, through various chemical processes. The amount of uric acid produced each day is determined by the breakdown of nuclear DNA (see below) and the levels of energy used, both of which are proportionate to the body size of the individual – a large person will produce more uric acid than a small person, for example. The concentration of uric acid in our bodily tissues depends also on the balance between the amount produced by the liver and the amount passed out via the kidneys. The ability of the kidneys to eliminate uric acid is determined to a great extent by inherited factors, as does the ability to clear uric acid from the blood and pass it out in the urine. Elimination of uric acid can also depend on the presence of other health problems, including kidney disease, and the type of medications taken.

In a healthy person, approximately two-thirds of the uric acid produced each day is passed out of the body in the form of urine. The remainder moves into the intestine and is broken down and eliminated in the faeces. When there is any excess uric acid it builds up in the bloodstream and is eventually deposited as urate crystals in the small joints and/or soft tissues.

Researchers have found that 75–90 per cent of people with gout have raised levels of circulating uric acid. Those with low levels suffer no apparent adverse effects.

How is uric acid (urate) produced in the body?

Many of the foods we eat contain chemicals called purines. Purines are nucleotides – that is, they are the basic molecular building blocks of DNA. Along with other nucleotides, purines are sources of energy that drive most of our bodily processes. After digestion, some purines are absorbed by the intestinal mucosa into nucleic acids. The others are rapidly degraded into uric acid. It is when the ability of the kidneys to eliminate uric acid (via the urine) is compromised that raised levels of uric acid occur – a condition known as hyperuricemia. 'Hyper' means increased, 'uric' refers to uric acid and 'emia' (sometimes spelt aemia) means blood. Thus hyperuricemia means raised levels of uric acid in the blood.

Raised levels of uric acid can be caused:

- when less uric acid is removed (via the kidneys) from the body than usual;
- when more is produced (by the liver) than normal;
- when both of the above occur.

Hyperuricemia

In testing for gout, the concentration of uric acid in the blood serum is measured and is a reflection of levels throughout the body. The recommended range of uric acid levels is less than 6 mg per 100 ml; the range of raised levels is 6–9 mg per 100 ml; and high levels are defined as more than 9 mg per 100 ml. Many people without gout have raised levels of uric acid, which is seen as an indication that the condition is liable to develop in them in future. Urate crystals take a long time to accumulate, and there may well be no symptoms whatsoever for months or even years – in fact about 95 per cent of people with hyperuricemia will remain symptom-free throughout their lives. On the other hand, a large study in the USA revealed that all participants with high concentrations of uric acid developed gout within four years.

In most cases of gout, there is no clear reason for the build-up of uric acid. However, it is known that certain factors can be responsible. These include:

- a high-purine diet
- poor kidney function or kidney disease
- being overweight
- high levels of fats (lipids) in the bloodstream
- high blood pressure (hypertension)
- regular, excessive alcohol consumption, or binge drinking
- the presence of certain diseases
- the use of certain medications
- inheritance of certain genes

Because gout was uncommon during and immediately after the First and Second World Wars, there is strong case for its still being referred to as 'the disease of plenty'. In fact, an acute attack often follows an evening of wining and dining or a holiday where restraint is set aside. The disorder is manifest typically in the overweight, hypertensive, overindulgent middle-aged or elderly male.

A high-purine diet

Gout arises from the normal breakdown of our own DNA into nucleic acids, then into purines, then into uric acid. This process accounts for some of the uric acid in our bodies, but a proportion of our purines comes from our diets as well – and again these purines are broken down into uric acid. Unfortunately, a diet that is high in purines burdens the kidneys with a large load for excretion. The same is the case in individuals who eat a large amount of food containing only a moderate amount of purines. The kidneys may not always be able to cope, hence the raised levels of uric acid.

Purines come from the nuclei of cells, not only of animals but also of plants. The foods that contain purines are: all meats, poultry and seafood, asparagus, mushrooms, dried peas and beans, lentils, soya, spinach and yeast. With meat, a good rule of thumb is that eating any part that has worked hard during its life is more likely to lead to raised levels of uric acid – liver and kidneys, for example. Chicken breast meat is also lower in purines than the legs on which the bird ran about. Active fish, such as sardines and salmon, contain more purines than such fish as plaice and flounder. Regarding alcohol, a product of yeast fermentation, the picture is a little more complex. Most alcoholic drinks contain only small amounts of purine, but its breakdown within the body causes uric acid levels in the blood to rise.

For people who consume moderate amounts of purine foods, cutting them out for five to seven days can significantly reduce levels of uric acid, as shown in a study in 1997[1]. People who are used to eating large amounts of purine foods can find by eliminating them for a few days that their uric acid levels fall even more. (There is more information about diet in Chapter 3.) A urine test after a week of elimination will show the extent of benefit that might be achieved from modifying the diet. If uric acid levels remain unchanged, purine intake is not the real problem. Purines are not the only cause of hyperuricemia – in fact, moderate to high purine consumption is thought to account for only 15 per cent of cases of gout.

Poor kidney function or kidney disease

Any disorder of the kidney reduces its ability to filter and eliminate uric acid. Whether kidney disease will produce hyperuricemia, however, depends to some extent on the concentration of uric acid in the blood prior to the onset of the disease. If the concentration was low and there was only a modest rise with the onset of disease, levels may remain within the normal range. If concentration was towards the upper end of normal, kidney disease is likely to lead to the development of hyperuricemia.

In cases where kidney disease is resolved and function returns to normal, uric acid levels may also return to normal. Of course, this depends also on the weight of the individual, their diet, alcohol intake and many other things.

Diseases of the kidney that can produce hyperuricemia are polycystic kidney disease, kidney disease due to lead poisoning in childhood and kidney disease due to excessive consumption of painkillers. Kidney disease in gout needs the specialized training of a rheumatologist.

Being overweight

Studies have shown that people who are overweight are more likely to have raised levels of uric acid in their blood than people who are not. In fact, being overweight is recognized as the most common cause of hyperuricemia. When weight is lost, the ability of the kidneys to pass out uric acid has been shown to improve. Also, uric acid in the blood reduces and high blood pressure can moderate. It can be seen, then, that weight has a significant impact on hyperuricemia and ultimately gout.

High levels of fats (lipids) in the bloodstream

The levels of fats in the blood are no higher in people with gout than in people with other diseases. However, it is thought that approximately half of the gout population have a condition called hypertriglyceridemia – raised levels of triglycerides in the blood (triglycerides are made up of glycerol and fatty acids). The main causes of raised triglyceride concentration in the blood are being overweight (eating a diet that is high in fats) and alcohol consumption, both of which are capable of raising levels of uric acid. Unfortunately, hypertriglyceridemia can lead to diabetes and heart disease, so should really be tackled. Correction of the cause of hypertriglyceridemia can lower levels of uric acid in the blood.

High blood pressure (hypertension)

Hypertension can reduce the kidney's ability to eliminate uric acid, which can in itself lead to hyperuricemia. Kidney disease can also be the cause of high blood pressure, which obviously compounds the situation. In addition, most of the diuretics (water tablets) prescribed to treat hypertension – frusemide and chlorothiazide for example – can lead to the development of hyperuricemia as a side effect. Spironolactone is the only diuretic that doesn't. The new ACE (angiotensin converting enzyme) inhibitors often successfully reduce high blood pressure, which in turn causes a lowering in levels of uric acid.

In people who are overweight, losing weight can also have the happy side effect of reducing high blood pressure. People with gout would be best advised to have their blood pressure taken at least once a year.

Regular, excessive alcohol consumption

There is a clear association between alcohol consumption and hyperuricemia. In fact after body weight it has the strongest correlation with levels of uric acid in the blood. Studies have shown higher than average concentrations of uric acid in individuals who drink more than two units of alcohol on a regular basis. They have also shown significant drops in concentration when the person cuts down on the amount they drink.

The presence of certain diseases

Any disease in which there is a rapid breakdown and turnover of bodily cells will raise levels of uric acid in the blood. In severe psoriasis, for example, the turnover of skin cells is much faster than normal. This has an effect on the degradation of purines, on the levels of uric acid produced and on the elimination of uric acid by the kidneys. Increased turnover of the bone marrow, in leukaemia and glandular fever for example, can also raise levels of uric acid.

Overweight diabetics with insulin resistance are at risk of developing hypertriglyceridemia (see above) and hyperuricemia because their uric acid is not effectively excreted by the kidneys. (Insulin resistance means the cells have difficulty converting glucose to energy. In an effort to compensate, the pancreas produces more insulin, which creates higher circulating levels of insulin than normal.) The result is often abnormal cholesterol and lipid levels, as well as weight gain. Raised levels of uric acid can also result from hypothyroidism (abnormally low activity of the thyroid gland) and disorders of the parathyroid glands (four small glands located behind the thyroid gland).

The use of certain medications

Diuretics (water tablets) prescribed for high blood pressure can lead to hyperuricemia. Also, chemotherapy drugs used to treat cancer often promote hyperuricemia due to the cell destruction they cause. Aspirin, in low doses, has the effect of reducing the excretion of uric acid, but in high doses it increases elimination. Aspirin should, therefore, be avoided if you suffer from gout. Because some other medications can cause hyperuricemia, check with your doctor to see if they can be the cause of your gout. An alternative medication may be available. If gout is the result of diuretic medication, stopping the diuretic may be possible and all that is required to return uric acid levels to normal.

Inheritance of certain genes

The genes a person inherits can promote either the overproduction or underproduction of uric acid. Small structural defects in the genetic code can affect the control mechanisms for the formation of uric acid, meaning the body produces an abnormally large amount of purine, the precursor to uric acid. The defective gene is located on the X chromosome, which relates to the male. As a result, only males suffer this particular defect, but it can be passed down by a female carrier who herself will either be mildly affected by hyperuricemia or completely normal. Alternatively, the genetic defect can arise spontaneously and there may be no other family members affected.

The ability of the kidneys to eliminate uric acid can also be passed down through families. The average rate of uric acid clearance is 10 ml per minute, the range being between 5 and 15 ml per minute. Those who inherit a clearance rate of only 5 or 6 ml per minute will obviously have much more difficulty eliminating a uric acid load than those who inherit a rate of 14 to 15 ml per minute. Apart from an inherited poor ability to excrete uric acid, the kidney is likely to be normal in all other respects.

The Arthritis Research Campaign (ARC) is sponsoring research to find out more about the underlying chemical and genetic processes that cause gout and also to search for more effective drugs to treat the disease. Much other research is under way.

When hyperuricemia is present

Hyperuricemia is the state of having raised levels of uric acid in the blood. Over a long period, the uric acid may become so concentrated that it can no longer stay dissolved, and tiny needle-like urate crystals accumulate in the synovial fluid of the joints (the thick lubricating liquid that is secreted into the joint). These urate crystals may, in turn, be present for several years without causing problems. Any of the following events may trigger an attack, however:

• an injury to the joint
• surgery
• illness

9

- an infection
- drinking too much alcohol
- increasing consumption of purine foods
- starvation
- dehydration
- increased stress
- use of drugs such as thiazides or, ironically, allopurinol, a long-term gout medication, when first used to lower uric acid levels

Where gout is concerned, there are a few exceptions to the rule. For instance, some people have high levels of circulating uric acid, but this is not accompanied by crystal formation and they do not experience gout. Also, rarely, some people with normal levels of uric acid do suffer from gout. In the main, though, the higher the level of uric acid, the greater the chance that crystals will form and be triggered into gout.

Topheous gout

In the case of an untreated sufferer who over a period of approximately ten years has experienced intermittent attacks of acute gout, a more chronic arthritis slowly develops in which symptoms will not completely resolve between attacks. The urate crystals responsible for acute attacks – which are generally only visible under a microscope – collect together beneath the skin to form a lump called a tophus. Tophi typically appear at the rim of the ear (where they are seen as small firm nodules), in the upper surfaces of the fingers, hands and feet and in the forearms and Achilles tendons. They can even grow in the kidney, severely compromising its filtering mechanisms (see below).

Topheous gout commonly causes deformity and joint immobility. In fact in the days before treatment was available, tophi could grow larger than a golf ball – particularly on the hands and feet – and render the individual unable to function. The tophi might even discharge a white chalky substance. (It is said that this was once used by some teachers to write on blackboards – what better example could there be of the grossness of gout in the past!) Furthermore, tophi would often become ulcerated and discharge blood and pus – and, of course, in this state they would be exceedingly painful. Thanks to modern medicines and knowledge about management techniques, today very few sufferers need be familiar with these extreme symptoms of the disease: only 15 per cent have tophi at all (compared with 50 per cent prior to the widespread use of medications that lower uric acid levels), and those who do will be prescribed life-long preventative medication that generally results in the tophi being reabsorbed into the body (see Chapter 2).

In other cases, tophi may drain spontaneously and become infected, further damaging the nearby joint. In elderly women who develop gout after taking diuretics or who suffer compromised kidney function, tophi may appear without previous history of acute gouty attacks. Also, a very rapid development of widespread tophi may occur in kidney and heart transplant patients who are treated with cyclosporine medication.

Topheous gout and kidney disease

When, in the past, no treatment was available for gout, tophi regularly formed in the body of the kidney and urate crystals in the collecting tubes. The cellular changes at the site of the tophi often led to kidney disease – and one result of that is high blood pressure. Of course, high blood pressure has always carried risks of its own, such as heart disease and further kidney disease. Kidney failure might eventually result. Fortunately, we now have medications that can generally prevent this state of affairs arising.

Kidney stones

The kidneys are highly implicated in gout because:

- when hyperuricemia is present, raised amounts of uric acid pass through the kidneys prior to being eliminated from the body, and
- the kidneys work hard to concentrate all the uric acid passing through them.

Because high levels of uric acid pass through the kidneys, tiny crystals of urate can collect together, accumulating into 'stones' that may reach more than 2.5 cm (1 inch) in diameter. In fact, experts believe that up to 40 per cent of gout patients have suffered a bout of renal colic due to the formation of a small stone (calculus) within the kidney or urinary tract. When stones remain in the kidney, a dull pain is a common symptom. However, when stones form in the ureters – the tubes that connect the kidneys to the bladder – the flow of urine can be blocked. A common symptom of this is blood in the urine – but sometimes the blood is not visible to the naked eye.

Urine analysis can show white blood cells, after which the patient may be sent for an X-ray or ultrasound scan. Kidney stones can be broken up by ultrasound waves and passed out with the urine, or extracted surgically. However, if levels of uric acid in the blood remain constant, further stones are likely to form.

Kidney stones can cause alarming symptoms. If you notice blood in your urine or start experiencing a constant dull or severe colicky pain in the kidney or groin area, you should visit your doctor immediately.

Paediatric gout

Gout is usually associated with the middle-aged male. Few people are aware that hyperuricemia can occur in individuals of any age. Even young children can develop the condition. In such cases the cause is generally a genetic purine and pyramidine enzyme deficiency. Purines and pyramidines are the building blocks of DNA (see p. 3). Like purines, pyramidines are broken down in the body by a specific enzyme. The first indications of problems may be crystals on the nappy or, in older children, in the urine. The medical term for paediatric gout is familial juvenile hyperuricemia nephropathy (FJHN); it was first described in 1962.

Recent studies have shown that some defects involving purine and pyramidine synthesis are genetic and thus could be seen in people of all ages and both sexes. If not treated adequately, disorders of purine and pyramidine synthesis can deteriorate so that ultimately dialysis is required. Indications of gout in children or adolescents should always be investigated as a matter of urgency.

Pseudogout

Gout-like attacks of pain, stiffness and swelling can be caused by deposits of calcium pyrophosphate crystals within the joints. This is called pseudogout, a form of arthritis which generally strikes at the elderly and immobile. The joints most commonly affected are the elbows, wrists, ankles, knees, fingers and toes, but the shoulder and hip joints are sometimes involved. In contrast, gout normally arises in a single joint, usually the base of the big toe.

Pseudogout can respond well to steroid injections and anti-inflammatory medication. However, it is important that the distinction between this type of arthritis and gout be made, as without the right treatment pseudogout can cause permanent joint damage.

There is no known way to prevent this disorder as its cause is unknown.

2

Getting Help From Your Doctor

If you think you are suffering from gout, it is important to secure a diagnosis as early as possible. Gout is one of the easiest forms of arthritis to treat. Remember that forming a close relationship with your doctor will be of benefit to you both – you will feel supported and understood and your doctor will have a better idea of the most suitable treatment options.

Preparing to see your doctor

If you are reading this book, you probably either suspect you have gout or you already have a diagnosis. For those who suspect, it may be helpful to know the official diagnostic criteria.

Diagnostic criteria

The American College of Rheumatology has defined the official criteria for the diagnosis of gout. Six or more of the following 11 criteria should be met to give a diagnosis:

- You must have suffered more than one acute attack of active arthritis.
- Maximum inflammation must develop within one day.
- You must have suffered at least one attack of oligoarthritis – a type of arthritis that affects children, linked with an eye disease called chronic iridocyclitis.
- Redness must be observed over the affected joint.
- The big-toe joint must be painful and/or swollen.
- Your first attack must be on the joint of one big toe, not on the joint of both big toes.
- An attack on the joints of only one ankle.
- There must be one or more tophi present.
- You must have hyperuricemia (raised levels of uric acid in the blood – see Chapter 1).
- You must have asymmetrical swelling within an affected joint on X-ray.
- There must be complete termination of an attack.

Be prepared for your doctor's questions

Your doctor's role is to look at your symptoms, ask a few questions, then attempt to fit the pieces together. Since certain other kinds of arthritis can mimic a gout attack – particularly acute septic arthritis or pseudogout – it is important that the right diagnosis be made. This also applies where an individual presents with a hot, painful and swollen toe, for example, as it could initially be taken for infection.

To properly assess your condition, your doctor may ask a series of questions. They are likely to include the following:

- Which areas of the body are involved?
- When did you first notice there was a problem?
- Did the pain come on suddenly or gradually?
- Was the pain worse during daytime or at night?
- Was the area hot, red and swollen?
- Did you experience other symptoms, such as fever, general achiness, loss of appetite, at the time the area became painful?
- Have you noticed lumps under your skin, especially on the ridge of the outer ear, the fingers, elbows, toes or around the Achilles tendon (connects the heel bone to the lower leg)?
- Have you ever had kidney stones?
- Does anyone in your family suffer from gout?

Give as much information as possible

To help point your doctor in the right direction, you should offer as much information as you can. Some details may be embarrassing, but they really should be disclosed.

- Your doctor must be reminded of any other illnesses you may have because gout can be associated with other health problems, for example kidney disease, high blood pressure, hypothyroidism, polycythaemia and psoriasis.

15

- You should state whether you were crash dieting or drinking large amounts of alcohol prior to an attack.
- Let your doctor know if you injured the area shortly before an attack. For example, did you stub your toe prior to it becoming swollen and painful?
- Let your doctor know if you had an infection prior to an attack.
- You should state whether you were eating more organ meat, shellfish or other foods high in purines than usual before the attack.
- Your doctor should also be reminded of any medications you take, as certain ones can trigger a gout attack. Examples are diuretics (water tablets) and low-dose aspirin.

Normally, doctors can diagnose gout on physical examination during an acute attack, combined with the individual's medical history. The definitive diagnosis of gout is dependent on finding uric acid crystals in the joint fluid during an attack (arthrocentesis – see below). Doctors can also administer a test, discussed in the next section, that measures the levels of uric acid in the blood. However, although uric acid levels are usually raised in individuals with gout, these levels alone are often misleading and may on measurement be normal or even low. The presence of raised levels of uric acid (hyperuricemia) increases the likelihood of the problem being gout. The development of tophi – often seen as small nodules on the ear – can confirm the diagnosis.

The blood test

In the blood test to measure levels of uric acid, blood is drawn from a vein or capillary. The laboratory then centrifuges the blood to separate the serum from the cells and the uric acid test is performed on the serum.

Preparing for the blood test

Your doctor may ask you to fast for four hours prior to the test. You may also be advised to stop taking any drugs that increase levels of uric acid. These include:

- aspirin
- caffeine
- alcohol
- diuretics (water tablets, such as Diamox, Burnex, Edecrin and Lasix)
- ascorbic acid (vitamin C tablets)
- diazoxide
- ethambutol
- methyldopa
- phenothiazines
- epinephrine
- cisplatin
- vincristine

Drugs that can decrease uric acid measurements should also, ideally, be temporarily discontinued prior to the test, with the backing of your doctor. These include:

- high-dose aspirin
- allopurinol
- clofibrate
- corticosteroids
- azathioprine
- guafenesin
- probenecid
- warfarin

The laboratory should be notified if you have recently undergone X-ray testing using contrast dyes. These chemicals increase uric acid levels in urine and decrease them in the blood.

Arthrocentesis

Because the blood test cannot give a definitive diagnosis, your doctor may wish to test the fluid in an affected joint, during an attack. If urate crystals are present the diagnosis is confirmed. This procedure is called arthrocentesis.

What happens during the procedure?

Your doctor will clean the area around the joint and may administer a local anaesthetic. A needle will then be inserted into the joint cavity and synovial fluid will be withdrawn. The doctor may then inject the joint with a drug that reduces inflammation, together with a painkiller. Slight pressure will then be applied to the place where the needle was inserted, and the doctor may wrap a bandage around it. The fluid will then be sent to a laboratory where it will be viewed under a microscope. If urate crystals are found, a diagnosis of gout can be confirmed.

Viewing under a microscope also allows the diagnosis of pseudogout, a similar condition described in Chapter 1, in which the joint pain is caused by deposition of pyrophosphate crystals. Pseudogout often attacks a different range of joints, such as the wrist, shoulder or knee.

What else will the doctor do?

Your doctor will also assess the following:

- your blood pressure;
- your kidney function;
- the levels of lipids (fats) in your blood;
- any existing medication, to gauge whether it has triggered the attack and to ensure it will not interact with any future gout medication;
- the need for X-rays of the affected joints if gout has been present for some time and not treated for any reason.

How is gout treated?

'The gout sir,' replied Mr Weller. 'The gout is a complaint as arises from too much ease and comfort. If you're ever attacked with the gout, sir, just you marry a widder as has got a good loud voice, with a decent notion of usin' it and you'll never have the gout again. It's a capital prescription, sir. I takes it reg'lar, and I can warrant it to drive away any illness as is caused by too much jollity.

Charles Dickens, *The Pickwick Papers*

This quote, funny as it may be, reflects the flawed reasoning that hindered progress in gout treatments for far too long. Fortunately, we have come a long way in the last hundred years and now have a great deal of knowledge about the condition. Currently, its treatment has three aims, which are to:

1 stop the current painful attack;
2 prevent further attacks by tackling the causes (such as high purine intake, drinking too much alcohol, being overweight, eating a high-fat diet);
3 if the above measures are not entirely successful, avert further attacks by using long-term preventative medications – joint damage, heart disease, kidney disease can be among the results if gout is not effectively treated.

Medications that treat an acute attack

When an attack of gout takes hold, all you will be able to think about is getting rid of the pain. Consequently, the first step in your treatment will focus on reducing the inflammation in the affected area. This should provide you with relief. Note that aspirin and its related drugs (salicylates) should be avoided as they can ultimately worsen gout.

Over-the-counter painkillers

Low-dosage codeine combined with paracetamol, available over the counter, can be of help to some people, as can ibuprofen, the only tablet-form non-steroidal anti-inflammatory drug available over the counter. Enteric-coated pills are easier on the stomach.

Prescription non-steroidal anti-inflammatory drugs (NSAIDs)

Acute gouty attacks are usually treated by prescription non-steroidal anti-inflammatory drugs. NSAIDs can calm the process that causes the inflammation, as a result of which the pain and swelling are eased. These drugs include naproxen sodium, indometacin and ibuprofen, the latter in a stronger dosage than available over the counter. NSAIDs are often prescribed in double the usual daily dose for the first two days, followed by regular recommended dosing for about one week, followed in turn by dosing that tapers down ultimately to discontinuation.

In the short term, dizziness, indigestion and nausea can arise with NSAID therapy, and prolonged usage can cause stomach and bowel irritation or aggravation of existing kidney disease. Taking NSAIDs with meals can reduce or eliminate these side effects. They should not be used where there is existing kidney disease, a peptic ulcer or inflammatory bowel disease. As there are approximately a hundred medications in this category, your doctor may want to see how you respond to different ones.

Cox-2 inhibitors

In recent years, Cox-2 inhibitors have been introduced. These offer a much lower risk of gastro-intestinal side effects than the traditional NSAIDs, with equal efficacy. In June 2002, the largest trial[2] for the treatment of gout was reported in the *British Medical Journal*, comparing indometacin (an NSAID medication) with the new Cox-2 inhibitor etoricoxib. The conclusion was that etoricoxib at 120 mg once a day provided the same rapid, effective relief as indometacin at 50 mg three times a day. This gives doctors a new choice for treating acute gout, so that gastro-intestinal upsets become less of a problem.

Colchicine

Colchicine is an old-fashioned remedy that was the first to be found effective in the nineteenth century. It is now prescribed mainly in cases where NSAIDs and Cox-2 inhibitors cannot be used. It is also used as a long-term preventative measure, preventing attacks in 80 per cent of patients – usually those with more modest elevations of uric acid in their blood. Unfortunately, this drug is slow to start working and may even cause abdominal pain, nausea and vomiting – but the side effects disappear once the patient stops taking the drug. Colchicine therapy is often given for 12 months or longer after uric acid levels are normalized. It can be prescribed in conjunction with life-long preventative medication that prohibits the build-up of uric acid in the blood.

Corticosteroids

These steroids may be prescribed when NSAIDs, Cox-2 inhibitors and colchicine are inappropriate or have failed, if infection is not present in the joint and only one or two joints are involved. Steroids can be injected directly into the joint or given via mouth. To inject into the joint will be a specialist decision.

Life-long preventative medications

The medications listed above can do nothing to prohibit the build-up of uric acid in the blood, nor can they prevent further acute attacks or stop urate crystals from accumulating in the joints. So what happens if the attacks continue (at the rate of three to four a year), if tophi are present, and if blood tests show that levels of uric acid are building up further? A low-purine diet, weight control, avoidance of alcohol and so on can successfully ward off additional attacks, but these measures don't always work – for example, where kidney disease is present or where medications must be taken for other health problems. Preventative treatment of hyperuricemia is expensive, life-long and carries a risk of toxic side effects. However, when all else fails, this is what your doctor will offer.

Life-long preventative medication works by normalizing levels of uric acid in the blood – in other words, correcting hyperuricemia. As a result, the attacks should stop and any tophi dissolve. (In some cases, medications fail to dissolve the tophi and they

21

must be removed surgically.) The resolution of hyperuricemia has the added bonus of improving the kidney problems that can accompany gout. It also means the prevention of the many complications to which hyperuricemia can lead.

Some people may think, 'Why bother making adjustments to my diet, losing weight, watching what I drink when preventative medications can be used instead?' It must be said that uric acid build-up in the first place is an SOS warning that something is very wrong. If you make no changes, continued weight gain can lead to high blood pressure, heart and lung disease, impaired kidney function, osteoarthritis; excess alcohol consumption can lead to serious liver damage; and a high-fat intake can lead to raised cholesterol levels and heart disease. Nor is this list exhaustive. Changing to healthier habits can prevent the diseases to which less healthy habits often lead. However, it's an unfortunate fact that taking one of the preventative medications can do nothing to improve the actual cause of the problem.

Because preventative medications are expensive and fail to tackle the underlying cause of hyperuricemia, they are generally offered to patients only in the following instances:

- if a health problem not in their control is causing their hyper-uricemia – such as kidney disease, psoriasis, hypothyroidism or leukaemia;
- if necessary medications affect uric acid levels in the blood;
- if they suffer from a purine synthesis disorder;
- if they appear to have inherited a genetic overproduction or underproduction of uric acid;
- if they have tried hard to alter their diet, lose weight etc. but have failed;
- if they suffer from an alcohol addiction.

Note that it is vital to let an acute attack settle down before embarking on one of the life-long medications. When the medications are taken erratically, flare-ups of gout are likely to ensue. It is important, therefore, that the medication be taken exactly as prescribed.

Allopurinol

The most common preventative treatment for gout is allopurinol. This drug works by inhibiting an enzyme – xanthine oxidase – that activates the production of uric acid by the liver. Taken daily over a long period, allopurinol will effectively reduce the levels of uric acid, then ensure that levels remain within normal boundaries. The usual starting dose is 100 mg daily, which is increased over the weeks according to the levels of uric acid. Most people end up taking 100–400 mg daily, the maximum daily dose being 800 mg. A dose of 300 mg is effective in 85 per cent of patients, however. The aim is to bring the levels of uric acid in the blood within the recommended range of less than 6 mg per 100 ml.

Allopurinol is known to be relatively safe, but all drugs have potential side effects. In 20 per cent of cases, usually when there is severe kidney disease, patients are hypersensitive to this drug and may develop a nasty rash, dermatitis and possibly liver dysfunction. In this instance, your doctor should be able to offer an alternative preventative medication.

Unfortunately, in some individuals gout attacks can become more frequent on commencement of a life-long treatment. To prevent this, an anti-inflammatory medication or colchicine may also be prescribed during the first three to six months of treatment.

If given at the time of an attack, allopurinol can prolong or worsen the situation. For this reason, at least a month should elapse after the attack before commencement of this type of treatment. Unfortunately, attacks may still occur in the first months of allopurinol therapy. In some cases, it may take as long as two years for urate crystals to be cleared. Note that if this type of medication is stopped, uric acid will accumulate again in the blood and urate crystals will once more form in the joints.

Uricosuric drugs

Uricosuric drugs such as probenecid and sulfinpyrazone lower the levels of uric acid in the blood by increasing its removal from the body via the kidneys (excretion). Like allopurinol, these drugs are a life-long commitment and need to be strictly adhered to. The side effects related to probenecid and sulfinpyrazone are not common or serious, but there is a risk of uric acid stone formation in the kidney during the initial treatment period, especially in individuals with pre-existing kidney disease. This risk can be minimized by drinking two to three litres of fluid a day.

If the first preventative treatment prescribed causes side effects, your doctor should be able to prescribe another type. Individuals with pre-existing disease or kidney stones should not be prescribed sulfinpyrazone.

The effects of probenecid are blocked by low-dose aspirin. Probenecid also inhibits the effectiveness of the drug heparin.

Where can I get more help and advice?

If you feel you need advice further to that given by your doctor, you can do the following:

- Your pharmacist may be able to offer more information on the lifestyle changes and medications that cause, treat and prevent gout.
- If a certain medication has been prescribed, read the patient information leaflet thoroughly. It will tell you how to use the medication and what benefits or possible side effects you can expect. Bear in mind, though, that many of the side effects listed are likely to be very rare indeed.
- Your doctor can put you in touch with a dietician if you need further assistance in adjusting what you eat. Alternatively, you can get help for any weight problems by joining one of the weight-loss organizations (see the Useful Addresses section for details).
- If alcohol addiction is a problem, it is recommended that you join a voluntary organization for help and support, such as Alcoholics Anonymous (AA). Your GP may be able to help you and also to advise you about local support groups.

3

Helping Yourself

When an acute attack of gout takes hold, all you will want to know is how to ease the pain. Your first step, if you are open to using medication, is to see your doctor and obtain a prescription for one of the non-steroidal anti-inflammatory drugs (NSAIDs), if they are appropriate to your case. It is advisable then to keep a supply of the drug handy for if and when further attacks occur.

The following guidelines can help ease the pain and reduce the longevity of the attack:

- Try to rest until the attack is over.
- Increase your fluid intake, trying to drink 3.5 litres (6 pints) of water a day. This should help flush out excess uric acid.
- Eat a bowl of cherries a day (see below).
- Try alternating hot compresses (for three minutes) and cold compresses (for 30 seconds) on the painful joint. You may wish to use gel packs, which can be heated in hot (not boiling) water or frozen in a freezer, and are available from some chemists. Alternatively, for hot compresses you could use a hot-water bottle. Make sure, whichever method you use, that the compress is not so hot as to burn the skin. A bag of frozen peas can also serve for cold compresses. This treatment sometimes helps to relieve the pain.
- Assuming you keep non-steroidal anti-inflammatory medications handy (these are effective at killing pain as well as at reducing inflammation), start taking the prescribed dosage – that is, if you wish to use drugs.
- Take belladonna for its anti-inflammatory properties, following the label dosage instructions. Belladonna can be purchased as an over-the-counter homeopathic remedy from chemists. A constitutional remedy prescribed by an experienced homeopath can help to reduce the likelihood of further attacks.

- Don't eat or drink anything you know is high in purines. If you tend to binge drink at the weekend, avoid it this time.
- Follow a therapeutic diet consisting mainly of cheese, milk, eggs and vegetables (excluding cauliflower, spinach, asparagus or mushrooms) for the duration of the attack.

If the factors that caused gout in the first place continue, an initial acute attack is likely to be followed, one or two years later, by further attacks. The intervals between flare-ups will become shorter and the attacks themselves more painful and debilitating as deposits of urate crystals form beneath the skin. While medications can be invaluable in treating an acute attack, they are not without side effects. The safest way to treat gout is, if at all possible, to make the necessary adjustments to your diet and lifestyle, so that raised levels of uric acid in the blood revert back to normal. However, if that is not possible for any reason, it is important that you don't be too hard on yourself. Fortunately, preventative medication is also available and it is far better than nothing at all. Stay positive and get on with enjoying a gout-free life.

How eating cherries can help

In 1950, a letter by Dr Ludwig W. Blau in *Prevention* magazine sparked off much interest in cherries for the treatment of gout. Dr Blau related how eating a bowl of cherries one day led to complete relief from his gout pain.[3] His gout had been so severe that he had been confined to a wheelchair – but after polishing off a bowl of cherries the pain in his foot had vanished by the next day. He continued eating a minimum of six cherries every day and was free of pain and able to get out of his wheelchair. Dr Blau's research resulted in many other gout sufferers being helped by the introduction of cherries into their daily diet. The same effect has also been reported with strawberries, leading nutritionists to conclude that these fruits contain an enzyme that helps to break down uric acid and facilitate its excretion from the body.

Look for fresh, raw cherries. Alternatively, frozen or canned unsweetened cherries or completely pure cherry juice may prove effective.

Correcting hyperuricemia

Before hyperuricemia can be tackled, you need to decide what is its probable cause. You can then make efforts to correct it. For example, if you are overweight you can help yourself by following a healthy eating plan that you know you stand a fair chance of continuing for the rest of your life (fad diets are not good for your body and can rarely be maintained). If you drink more than two standard drinks of alcohol a day, you can help yourself by cutting down to healthier levels. If hypertension is also a problem, control of the above factors may have the happy outcome of reducing blood pressure and the need for diuretics (water tablets).

A common problem in gout is that several factors may have worked together to cause hyperuricemia. A typical gout sufferer might be an overweight, middle-aged male who is a regular alcohol drinker, eats meat twice a day and has raised levels of fats in his blood (hypertriglyceridemia – see Chapter 1). Since his friends may share the same lifestyle, it can be extremely difficult to find the motivation to make changes. I suggest that if this description fits you, you enlist the support of your family and friends, impressing on them that your gout will worsen if you don't make changes and that the only alternative is to take medication for the rest of your life.

When levels of uric acid have been normal for about a year, gout attacks will either become mild and infrequent or disappear altogether.

Stabilizing medication

While you are attempting to normalize levels of uric acid in your blood, you may wish to take medication to reduce the risk of further flare-ups of gout. The best ones are probably colchicine and NSAID drugs – your doctor will know which is more suitable. Then, as you attempt to correct your hyperuricemia, your blood serum should be checked regularly by your doctor.

Knowing that levels of uric acid are falling should give you that extra boost to help you on your way. When you have suffered no attacks of gout for 12 months, it should be safe to come off the medication and continue as you mean to go on.

Note that it is vital to do nothing either to lower or to raise your levels of uric acid during an attack, or while there is persistent gouty inflammation. Any deviation from the norm – barring recommended medication – can worsen the attack.

Reducing dietary purines

If you normally consume large amounts of dietary purines, cutting down can have a substantial effect on the levels of uric acid in your blood. On the other hand, if you consume only moderate amounts of purine, your uric acid levels are likely not to alter very much on cutting down. In that case, other factors will have led to your hyperuricemia and you need not alter your intake of purines. Only people who eat large amounts of purines should try to reduce their purine foods. Alternative sources of protein should be included in a low-purine diet. These could include, for example, tofu, tempeh and miso.

Since many protein foods contain purine, it is recommended that your intake of protein should not exceed 100 g (3 oz) per day. (Many people in whom hyperuricemia is diagnosed are found to eat large amounts of protein in the form of meats – hence the high level of purines.) As a guide, a portion of 100 g of meat contains 25 g protein; of pasta 12 g; of rice 8 g. One thick slice of wholemeal bread contains 3 g protein.

The following is a list of foods showing their relative purine contents:

Very high purine content: Organ meats such as liver, kidney, brains, heart and sweetbreads
Game meats such as rabbit, venison, pheasant, duck, goose and partridge

High purine content: Vegetables such as spinach, asparagus, cauliflower and mushrooms
Chicken
Fish such as herring, sardines, scal-

lops, mackerel, roe, shrimp, mussels and anchovies

Yeast (baker's and brewer's) and yeast extracts (Marmite and Vegemite for example)

Meat extracts and gravies, broth and consommé)

Beer, wines and spirits

Dried peas and beans

Moderate purine content: Oatmeal, peas, beans and other legumes, lentils, soya, spinach, tripe and wholemeal (also called wholewheat or wholegrain) bread and pasta

Beef and pork

The foods recommended in gout are:

Breads, especially white bread and crackers (limit intake of higher-fat foods such as muffins, French toast, biscuits and doughnuts, and also of wholemeal bread and biscuits – see above)

Cheese (all kinds in moderation, and preferably low-fat)

Cereals and cereal products (all kinds except oatmeal)

Eggs (in moderation)

Fruit juices (all kinds)

Fruit (all kinds; avocado in limited quantities)

Gelatin

Ice cream

Milk (fat-free and low-fat)

Noodles

Nuts

Oils (all oils, in limited quantities)

Pasta (wholemeal pasta in moderation)

Potatoes (limit intake of higher-fat forms such as chips, potato crisps and creamed potatoes)

Soups (cream soups should be made with low-fat milk)

Vegetables (except spinach, asparagus, cauliflower and mushrooms)

White rice

Eating healthily

Unfortunately, removing purines from the diet is known to cause a drop in uric acid levels of only 15 per cent. Healthy eating can reduce levels further; it will have the happy side effect of weight loss in people who are overweight, and it can reduce levels of triglycerides (fats) in the blood. Healthy eating can also reduce high blood pressure and the risk of both heart and kidney disease. It can therefore be of great benefit in gout.

Although it may be difficult at first to make the recommended changes, the benefit to your overall health will make the effort worthwhile. However, if you find you are unable to make great changes, don't feel guilty or despondent. Small changes are better than no changes at all – they will make a difference. Healthy eating advice is given in Chapter 4.

Reducing alcohol consumption

An individual's alcohol consumption is strongly linked to levels of uric acid in the blood, someone drinking moderate to high amounts of alcohol being far more likely to develop hyperuricemia than someone who doesn't drink, or drinks very little. Studies have shown that people who consume more than two units of alcohol on a regular basis have higher than average concentrations of uric acid in the blood. Obviously, some people drink rather more than two units, which has a knock-on effect on levels of uric acid.

Alcohol causes a rise in uric acid levels for the following reasons:

- The metabolism of alcohol creates a chemical called lactate, which reduces the elimination of uric acid by the kidneys.
- Certain properties of alcoholic drinks can pile on the pounds – in males it is generally around the middle – and carrying excess weight has its own links with hyperuricemia.
- Many alcoholic beverages contain purines.

Quite often people don't realize the extent of their alcohol consumption, especially if they tend to drink a glass of wine or two with meals, then more at night socially, or while watching the TV. Drinking beer or lager socially at the pub is a way of life for many people, but they rarely count the number of pints they drink in a week. A person who abstains all week but drinks several pints of beer at the weekend is just as likely to have raised levels of uric acid as someone who drinks beer almost every night. It can be difficult to break what is often a social habit, but it should not be necessary to abstain from alcohol altogether. Try drinking more slowly and replace some of your alcoholic drinks with non-alcoholic ones. Ask your doctor to measure your uric acid levels after cutting down for a while, then decide whether you need to cut down further.

People who binge drink or drink regular amounts of alcohol tend to be overweight. This transpires because of the effect of the kilojoules in the alcohol. Cutting down, therefore, is another great way to lose weight.

Fluids

To reduce the risk of uric acid crystallizing in the joints (the cause of the severe pain in acute gout) it is important to drink plenty of fluids, obviously not including alcohol. Ideally, you should try to drink as much as 3.5 litres (6 pints) of water a day. It is fine to include other fluids in this amount, such as fruit juices and herbal teas. However, as caffeine can stress adrenal glands that are overworked in any case where disease is present, it should be consumed in moderation, if at all.

A problem for many is finding an acceptable alternative to caffeine. Coffee, tea, cocoa and cola drinks can be replaced by fruit and vegetable juices and herbal teas – green tea is very good, as is rooibosch (redbush) tea.

If you are trying to lose weight, bear in mind that many soft drinks contain large amounts of sugar and should be avoided.

4
Eating to Combat Gout

Being overweight appears to be the most common determining factor for excess uric acid production. Not all people with raised levels of uric acid, and ultimately gout, are overweight – as we have seen, kidney disease or genetic predisposition are two other causes of overproduction. However, it can safely be stated that the majority of gout sufferers are overweight to some degree, as several recent studies have shown. Losing weight should, therefore, be a priority – but avoid crash dieting as it can be counter-productive, increasing uric acid levels and causing an acute attack. Ideally, you should aim to lose no more than two pounds a week.

When a person with gout begins to lose weight, they are, for the following reasons, mounting a two-pronged attack on the cause of their disorder:

- The kidneys are more able to eliminate uric acid.
- In some cases, the production of uric acid by the liver is reduced.

Weight loss can also have the happy effect of moderating blood pressure. Obviously the risk of developing the disorders that high blood pressure can lead to is then much reduced.

How can I lose weight?

Starving yourself is not recommended as a means of parting with the pounds; neither is fad dieting where entire nutritional components are cut out, such as a carbohydrate-restricted diet, the 'cabbage-soup diet' and so on. It is important to choose a diet that is sustainable, which means eating a wide variety of healthy foods. Happily, changing to healthy eating will naturally cause weight loss in gout sufferers who are overweight; it will reduce levels of lipids (fats) in the blood; and it can reduce raised blood pressure.

However, it is essential that you *slowly* retrain your palate to accept different tastes. For this reason, it is advisable to cut back gradually on the amounts of sugar, salt and saturated fat you consume. It takes only 28 days of eating a food regularly for it to become a habit.

Keeping a diary

Keeping a food-intake diary is an excellent way of monitoring your progress. I suggest that you buy a notebook and devote a page to each day, listing all the foods you eat – including snacks and drinks.

Goals

It's a good idea to set goals on the very first page. For example, you may wish to make a goal of eating two types of vegetables each day. Without the diary, you may assume you have done badly – but upon reading your entries you may see that you've actually eaten two types of vegetables three or four times a week. That's a good starting point. Now you can focus on slowly increasing that amount.

As time goes by and you begin to achieve your goals as a matter of habit, list a new set of slightly more difficult ones.

Examples of long-term, general healthy eating goals are as follows:

- to eat two or three types of vegetables every day;
- to eat two or three portions of fruit every day;
- to eat nuts, seeds and dried fruit as snacks once or twice a day;
- to drink as much as 3.5 litres (6 pints) of water a day, including that in fruit and vegetable juices and green tea;
- to use vegetable oil, flower oil, corn oil or olive oil in cooking and dressing (extra virgin olive oil is best, and hemp oil, which is very nutritious, is also great for dressings);
- to minimize the amount of salt added to cooking and baking, and to avoid sprinkling it on food at the table;

- to reduce your intake of meat and dairy products, making sure to spread butter very thinly;
- to cut down on caffeine – coffee, chocolate, cola drinks, tea and cocoa;
- to cut down on alcohol (seek your doctor's advice if cutting down is a problem);
- to cut down on saturated fats;
- to cut down on table sugar and other sugar-containing products, such as cakes, sweets, biscuits and sugar-coated cereals;
- to cut out junk food;
- to cut out artificial sweeteners;
- to cut out fried foods (but see p. 40).

The reasons why many of the above foods should be minimized or cut out are explained later in this chapter. I will just add that if you are ultimately unable to eliminate certain foods, don't be discouraged. Reducing your intake should have a positive effect on your weight and the levels of uric acid in your blood. Ask your doctor to check your levels after changing your eating habits for a month or so – an indication that there is already less uric acid in your blood may give you an added incentive to persevere with your diet.

Help with cutting down

Changing the habits of a lifetime may be the hardest thing you have ever done, but for the sake of your health it is worth the effort. The following pointers may help you on your way:

- Eat one biscuit instead of two and cut yourself a smaller slice of cake prior to more drastically minimizing, or eliminating, foods containing sugar. If you find you are craving sugar, remember that the lift it offers will be brief – the next effect being a plummet into a low mood. Staving off hunger with fruit (fresh and dried), nuts and seeds is not only a far healthier choice, it also stabilizes blood-sugar levels, helping to ward off the low mood.

- Reduce your intake of caffeine products very gradually. Withdrawing too fast may cause fatigue and headaches.
- When drinking socially, order half pints of beer instead of pints, or drink alcohol-free wine, beers and lagers. Remember, it should not be necessary to eliminate alcohol entirely, unless you have an addiction to it of course. In this event, you would be best advised to enlist the help of your doctor or a local Alcoholics Anonymous group.
- Stock fresh foods.
- Get into the habit of snacking on a variety of nuts, such as almonds, cashews, walnuts, Brazils and pecans; dried fruit, such as raisins, dates and apricots; and even seeds, such as pumpkin, hemp, sesame and sunflower. These should not spoil your appetite for an upcoming meal. Obviously, if you suffer from a nut allergy, leave nuts alone.
- Select a salad instead of fries when eating out.
- Slowly increase the number and variety of fruits and vegetables you use.
- Gradually reduce the amount of salt you add to your food and in cooking, especially if high blood pressure is already a problem. Remember that salt is commonly used as a preservative and added to most processed, pre-packaged foods. Rock salt and sea salt are healthier alternatives, but should still be used sparingly.
- Eat three or four small meals a day, with some snacks in between.
- Never go more than two to three hours without eating – which means you should never go hungry. This will help control your blood-sugar levels.
- Don't skip breakfast. After fasting during the night, the body requires the glucose obtained from foods. Studies have shown that when a meal is missed, brain function can be compromised.
- Avoid missing other meals. When we allow ourselves to become very hungry, the sugary, high-fat foods that are bad for us become more tempting.
- Listen to your body. Stop eating when you feel satiated.

Overeating creates a large mass of undigested food, and many associated problems.

- Don't mistake thirst for hunger. As the body's thirst mechanism is poorly developed, determine whether you really are hungry and don't simply need a drink.
- Don't use your stomach as an emotional rubbish bin. Try to find other outlets for your feelings, such as yoga, pilates and t'ai chi.
- Relax for at least ten minutes before starting each meal. Don't rush off straight after eating.
- Eat unhurriedly and chew thoroughly. Enjoy your food.
- At least half of your calorie intake should be made up of complex carbohydrates (see p. 43). These include fruits, vegetables and grains such as couscous and brown rice.
- Fats (oils) should be an important part of your diet. *Unsaturated* fats (also known as polyunsaturated fats) are greatly beneficial to health. These include olive, safflower, sunflower and corn oils. *Saturated* fats are largely derived from animals and should be consumed in moderation, if at all. Examples are lard, suet, butter and dripping.
- If you are trying to reduce your intake of purines, remember to replace them with sufficient protein foods.
- Eat plenty of fibre in the form of fruits, vegetables, breads, cereals and legumes (not dried peas and beans).
- Try not to shop when you feel hungry. You won't then be so tempted to buy the less healthy foods.
- Drink as much water as possible, particularly during a flare-up of gout.
- Try to exercise regularly. You can lose weight more successfully when you exercise and cut down food intake.
- Try to avoid stress. Gout is often triggered during or after a particularly stressful time.

So exactly what foods should I eat?

Dr John McDougall, a prominent promoter of hygienist and naturopath health principles, recommends that his gout patients follow a low-fat diet with no animal products whatsoever. He also advises that they eliminate highly allergenic plant foods such as wheat, corn and citrus fruits, claiming that benefits will be seen within a few days. He believes that the things we eat can cause arthritic disease by contributing to the formation of 'complexes' within the immune system – complexes acting much like slivers of wood stuck under the skin, causing severe inflammation of the joints.[4] Most doctors are of a less radical persuasion, however, recommending that their patients cut down on purine foods and monitor the effects. It is only when gout flare-ups persist regardless of your efforts that you should maybe try to cut out animal products altogether and, if that fails, cut out wheat, corn and citrus fruits, as Dr McDougall recommends – these plant foods are widely recognized as having allergenic properties and being of some detriment to people with arthritic disease. Of course, if you would prefer to follow his recommendations at the outset, good for you. You should soon know whether your diet was the problem.

From the previous chapter you may now have an idea that you should eat lots of fruit, vegetables, grains and nuts. The following short sections should clarify the foods you would be best advised to cut down on and those that are better for you. I will just add that the World Health Organization recommends that we each consume five portions of fruit and five portions of vegetables a day. As ten portions is a lot for most people to achieve, I suggest that you try to eat a total of at least five portions a day in some combination of fruit and vegetables. Each of the following is equivalent to one portion:

- 100 g ($3\frac{1}{2}$ oz) of a very large fruit such as melon or pineapple
- one large fruit such as orange, banana or apple
- two medium fruits, such as kiwi fruits, plums or satsumas
- 100 ml ($3\frac{1}{2}$ fl oz) freshly squeezed fruit or vegetable juice
- 100 g ($3\frac{1}{2}$ oz) berries or cherries
- a large bowl of salad
- 90 g (3 oz), cooked weight, green vegetables

- 80 g ($2\frac{3}{4}$ oz), cooked weight, root vegetables such as carrot or swede – don't include potatoes, sweet potatoes or yams
- 70 g ($2\frac{1}{2}$ oz), cooked weight, small vegetables such as peas or sweetcorn
- 80 g ($2\frac{3}{4}$ oz) pulses, such as lentils

Reducing sugar and refined carbohydrates

In his research, Professor John Yudkin observed that people with gout eat far more sugar than others. He then discovered that sugar actually increases the amount of uric acid in the blood, which gives us yet another cause of the development of gout. Unfortunately, our diets today are often high in sugar and refined carbohydrates, such as biscuits, cakes and pastries. Sugar contains no nutritional value at all. In fact, sugar consumption has been linked with many disorders, from diabetes to heart disease and cancer. You probably know that sugar converts into energy. What you may not know is that we can actually obtain all the sugars and energy we need from fruit and complex (unrefined) carbohydrates, such as grains and lentils, which convert into sugar in the body as nature intended.

Reducing salt

Salt is commonly used as a preservative and added to most processed, pre-packaged foods – cornflakes, for example, are high in salt. As a result, people who eat a lot of processed foods may be consuming more salt than they realize, especially when that used in cooking and at the table is taken into account. Try using herbs and spices for flavouring, but in moderation. Sea salt contains more minerals than ordinary salt, but it is still salt – so use sparingly.

Reducing meat and dairy produce

It is only people who eat large amounts of purines who should try to reduce their purine intake. Red meat, particularly offal, and shellfish contain perhaps the highest levels. You should, therefore, try to eat a piece of offal meat weighing about 85 g (3 oz), or the size of the palm of your hand, no more than twice a week.

If you then suffer a flare-up of gout, it would obviously be best to cut out offal and shellfish completely. Poultry and fish are good sources of protein and oils, but they do contain purines. Limit your consumption of the fish high in purines, such as herring, sardines, scallops, mackerel, roe, shrimp, mussels and anchovies, and eat poultry no more than twice a week. If, after doing this, you continue to suffer attacks of gout, you would be well advised to eliminate all meats, poultry and fish from your diet, replacing them with other forms of protein, such as tofu, tempeh, and miso.

Meat and dairy products contain arachidonic acid, a fatty acid that contributes to the inflammation experienced in arthritic conditions. In one study,[5] arthritis sufferers reported a complete absence of symptoms after following a fat-free diet for seven weeks. Interestingly, when fats were reintroduced into their diets their symptoms returned. It is recommended, therefore, that people with gout cut down on the amount of meat and dairy produce they eat, whether purine intake appears to be the cause of their hyperuricemia or not.

Reducing the wrong sort of fats

Fats (fatty acids) are the most concentrated sources of energy in our diet, one gram of fat providing the body with nine calories of energy. However, as you may be aware, some fats are beneficial to health, while others are capable of raising cholesterol levels. They can also cause a condition called hypertriglyceridemia, which is a causal factor in gout.

Fats can be categorized as follows:

• *Saturated fat* Believed to be implicated in the development of heart disease, saturated fat comes mainly from animal sources and is generally solid at room temperature. Although margarine was, for many years, believed to be a healthier choice over butter, nutritionists have now revised their opinion, for some of the fats in the margarine hydrogenation process are changed into trans-fatty acids, which the body metabolizes as if they were saturated fatty acids – the same as butter. Butter is a valuable source of oils and vitamin A, but should be used sparingly. Margarine, on the other hand, is an artificial product containing many additives.

- *Unsaturated fat* Unsaturated fat, including polyunsaturated fat and monounsaturated fat, has a protective effect on the heart and other organs. Omega 3 and omega 6 oils occur naturally in oily fish, nuts and seeds, and are usually liquid at room temperature. Because there is recent evidence that a relative increase in consumption of unsaturated fats from nuts and oils can help to lower levels of uric acid, even with a relatively high intake of protein, it is recommended that people with gout use cold-pressed oil (olive, rapeseed, hempseed, safflower and sunflower oil) daily, for dressings and in cooking. Extra virgin olive oil is best suited to cooking, however, as it suffers less damage from heat than other oils.

I must add that the process of frying changes the molecular structure of foods, rendering them potentially damaging to the body. If you must fry something, it is best to use a small amount of extra virgin olive oil and to cook at a low temperature. A healthier alternative is to sauté in a little water or tomato juice, or to grill, bake and steam. Stir-frying is good – but by this I mean cooking the food in a little *water* and just drizzling on olive oil afterwards. If you love chips, coat thick slices of potato with olive oil before baking in the oven. They're not only healthier this way, they taste better too!

Eggs

You are no doubt aware that eggs are high in cholesterol, which is a type of fat. However, they also contain lecithin, a superb biological detergent capable of breaking down fats so that they can be utilized by the body – very useful for people with gout. Lecithin also prevents the accumulation of too many acid or alkaline substances in the blood and encourages the transportation of nutrients through the cell walls. Eggs should be soft-boiled or poached – a hard yolk will bind the lecithin, rendering it useless as a fat-detergent.

Fresh fruit and vegetables

Try to eat as much fruit and vegetable as possible – but only small amounts of asparagus, mushrooms and cauliflower, which are high in purines. Make a variety of salads and try to eat one every day. When you cook vegetables, boil them in the minimum of unsalted (or lightly salted) water for the minimum amount of time. Lightly steaming or stir-frying (as above) are healthy alternatives.

Legumes (peas and beans)

Because all peas and beans contain moderate amounts of purines, try to limit the amount you eat. The soya bean and soya products, such as soya milk, tofu, tempeh and miso, also contain purines (see below), so should also be eaten in moderation.

Nuts

Nuts, on the other hand, should be an intrinsic part of your diet. All nuts contain vital nutrients, but almonds, cashews, Brazils and pecans perhaps offer the greatest array. Eat a wide assortment as snacks, with cereals and in baking.

Grains

Wheat is our staple grain in the west, refined wheat flour the product with which most of our cakes, pastries, biscuits and breads are made. However, wheat (and corn, to a lesser extent) is known to be particularly acid-forming, and people with gout would be well advised to limit the amount of wheat products they eat. More beneficial grains are oats, barley, bran, brown rice, couscous, millet, rye, spelt and quinoa. These are all excellent sources of protein, complex carbohydrates (see below), fibre, vitamins and minerals. Try eating rice cakes, oatmeal biscuits and cake, carob cake, scones (made with ground rice) and carrot cake (made with brown-rice flour).

Now that we have established what foods we ought to be eating, it's time to think about how we might combine them, in the right proportions, to arrive at a healthily balanced diet geared to gout. Depending on how active you are, you should be eating in total between 1,800 and 3,000 calories a day. The following sections should help you achieve that intake in the right balance. I also offer advice on food combining and supplements, followed by suggested menus to get you started.

Protein

Many protein foods are high in purines, which we know are a problem in gout. Many experts recommend, therefore, that the intake of protein should not exceed 25 per cent of your total calorie intake per day. I know it is difficult to judge the exact amount of a particular food in your diet. However, if you at least try to consume the recommended amounts of meat, as well as fruit, vegetables, nuts, seeds, legumes, soft-boiled egg yolks, soya products and so on, you will be in the right region. Remember, too, that you can lower your levels of uric acid even if you are not able to follow this diet to the letter. Try to do the best you can and appreciate the fact that you are helping your body to fight this disease.

One study into the value of reducing protein in gout has suggested that eating tofu, which is made from the soya bean and is a source of complete protein, is a better choice than meats. However, soya products do contain purines, albeit in lesser amounts than meat, so should not be consumed every day. There are many soya bean products, including soya milk, tofu, tempeh and miso. Tofu is particularly versatile and can be used in both savoury and sweet dishes (see the Further Reading section for details of an excellent soya cookbook).

If you find that you are eating considerably less than the recommended amount of protein, I strongly advise that you take free-form amino acids, which are available from healthfood shops. The herb acidophilus is also useful, taken twice a day.

Recommended protein consumption

The following measurements should give you a rough idea not only of your protein intake, but also of your total calorific consumption (examples of carbohydrate and fat calories are given later in this chapter). Use them in conjunction with the recommended proportion of protein intake within total calorie intake that was noted above (25 per cent).

Here are the calorific values of some common protein foods:

- 28 g (1 oz) grilled haddock – a very small piece – yields 40 calories;
- 28 g (1 oz) roasted chicken – also a very small piece – yields 40 calories;
- 28 g (1 oz) cottage cheese yields 15 calories;
- 28 g (1 oz) Parmesan cheese yields 120 calories;
- 28 g (1 oz) soya bean yields 50 calories;

Butter, which contains some protein, is very high in fat – 28 g (1 oz) of butter contains 226 calories. I reiterate, therefore, that butter should be used very sparingly.

Carbohydrates

Our digestive systems break down carbohydrates into simple sugars that are used to fuel essential body processes such as brain function, nervous system function and muscle activity. In short, we obtain vital energy from carbohydrate-containing foods. A word of warning, however: any excess carbohydrate is converted to fat by insulin, the 'fat-storage' hormone.

To ensure that fats and proteins are effectively broken down, and to guarantee the production of sufficient energy, we need to eat plenty of what are known as complex carbohydrates. These include fruit, vegetables and grains (breads, pasta, brown rice, cereals, couscous, millet, barley, bulgar wheat and other cereals). On the other hand, so-called simple carbohydrates will only pile on the pounds and cause levels of uric acid to rise. They include table sugar and the sugars found in sweets, cakes, biscuits and sweetened cereals. The sugar in these foods causes erratic fluctuations in blood-sugar levels – meaning that after consuming them you will experience a spurt of energy, followed by a dip into a low mood. Here we have yet another reason why simple carbohydrates should be avoided as much as possible. Try to snack on a variety of fruit and nuts instead of cakes and biscuits. If you are persistent, you should soon lose that urge for sweet foods.

Recommended carbohydrate consumption

Remember that we should all try to eat at least five portions of fruit and vegetables a day. We can go some way towards meeting that target just by eating enough of the right sort of carbohydrates. For people with gout it is recommended that 55 per cent of their daily calorific intake be in the form of carbohydrate. If you are trying to lose weight, here are the calorific values of some recommended sources of complex carbohydrates:

- 28 g (1 oz) banana yields 22 calories;
- 28 g (1 oz) orange yields 12 calories;
- 28 g (1 oz) apple yields 17 calories;
- 28 g (1 oz) wholemeal pasta yields 35 calories;
- 28 g (1 oz) wholemeal bread yields 38 calories;
- 28 g (1 oz) cabbage yields 4 calories.

Do bear in mind that wholemeal foods are moderately high in purines and have allergenic properties (see pp. 29 and 41), and should therefore be eaten in moderation.

Fats and oils

As already noted, fats (fatty acids) are the most concentrated sources of energy in our diet. Foods containing good (unsaturated) fat – omega 3 and omega 6 – are crucial to good health (see p. 40). Oils are also a natural source of vitamin E, which is an important antioxidant. (Antioxidants mop up damaging 'free radicals' that build up in the cells of the body and are part of any disease process.) However, remember that saturated fat, when consumed regularly, can lead to the development of heart disease. Eating fried foods is not recommended for people with gout – grill your food instead.

Recommended unsaturated fat consumption

It is estimated that most adults consume approximately 42 per cent of their total daily calories as fat – most of it saturated.

However, the recommended daily intake is 20 per cent. Eating the necessary unsaturated fats will ensure reduced calorie intake and greater energy provision. It will also reduce the risk of developing hypertriglyceridemia (see Chapter 1).

Here are the calorific values of some fat-containing foods:

- 28 g (1 oz) oil yields 130 calories;
- 28 g (1 oz) butter yields 226 calories;
- 28 g (1 oz) egg yields 80 calories;
- 28 g (1 oz) oily fish yields 60 calories.

Fibre (roughage)

Fibre, formerly known as roughage, is the indigestible part of plants. It is the cellulose fibres forming the leaf webbing in green vegetables, the skins of sweetcorn and beans, and the husks of wheat and corn. Fibre – a type of carbohydrate – is found in fruits, vegetables, nuts, seeds, beans, peas, lentils, wholemeal breads and cereals (wheat, oats, rye, barley, quinoa, spelt, buckwheat, corn and so on).

It is estimated that people in the West consume only 12 g (under $\frac{1}{2}$ oz) of fibre on average per day, instead of the recommended 20–30 g (1 oz or under). However, the latter amount was, in fact, consumed up to the time of the Second World War. Fibre is useful not only because of its high nutritional value, but also because it is a bulking agent that quickly sweeps the bowel clean, ensuring no unhealthy waste products lurk in hidden corners.

When waste products persistently linger in the bowel, as occurs in low-fibre diets, toxins are absorbed back into the blood stream causing eventual weakening of the immune system. The slower and more regulated absorption of glucose into the bloodstream is also aided by fibre – as a consequence of which the individual avoids plummeting into hunger troughs and craving sugar to raise blood-sugar levels. Another advantage of fibre is that the appetite is satiated on comparatively fewer calories. All in all, fibre is an essential food component and crucial to improved health.

The only form of fibre you may wish to cut down on is wheat. This cereal is a common allergen (see p. 37), and because it is acid-forming it can contribute to raised levels of uric acid in the blood.

Food combining

Many foods are not easily digested when eaten together. The Hay system of food combining recommends, for example, that high-protein foods (such as meats, dairy produce, eggs, fish, nuts and soya) should not be eaten at the same meal as high-carbohydrate foods (such as rice, potatoes and bread) because proteins require an acid medium in the stomach to be broken down whereas carbohydrates require an alkaline medium. This means that the bulk of the diet should be fruits, salad and vegetables, as these are not high in either carbohydrate or protein.

Some people with arthritic disease, including gout, have claimed to feel much better within a few days of commencing a food combining diet. (For details of the Hay system of food combining, see the Useful Addresses section.)

Food supplements

When an individual is in a state of dis-ease, their nutritional requirements are increased for various reasons. There is thus a strong case for taking good quality food supplements in a sensible manner. However, steer clear of vitamin A supplementation as it is believed to increase the risk of gout attacks.

The following supplements are recommended in gout:

Pantothenic acid and vitamin B complex

In order to excrete uric acid, the body needs sufficient of the B vitamins, particularly pantothenic acid – also known as vitamin B_5. This vitamin is crucial for the production of the anti-stress hormones, the release of energy from protein, carbohydrates, fats and sugars, and for good health of the nervous system. It is interesting to note that gout often follows times of stress, and stress depletes the body of the B vitamins. This may be the reason why gout sufferers are typically deficient in the B vitamins and why supplementation can be useful.

The suggested dosage of pantothenic acid for gout treatment is 500 mg twice daily, one dose taken with breakfast and one with the evening meal. Follow the label dosage instructions for the B complex vitamins.

Vitamin C

One of the more potent antioxidants, vitamin C is very much the main stress vitamin, and is probably the most important nutrient for immune system function. One study found that pain was significantly reduced in elderly people with arthritis and gout when vitamin C was added to their diet.

Cod liver oil

Recent research has strongly suggested that the age-old belief that cod liver oil is good for the joints is true. A study in Cardiff[6] found that cod liver oil might delay or even reverse the destruction of joint cartilage and inflammatory pain associated with joint disease. Make sure that you purchase the variety containing EPA and DHA – fish oil concentrates – since it is probably more effective. Follow the instructions on the label.

Glucosamine

Glucosamine is a promising treatment for all types of arthritic pain (including gout) and is backed by a number of double-blind, placebo-controlled studies. In these studies, glucosamine, often combined with chondroitin, has been shown to rehabilitate cartilage, reduce the progression of osteoarthritis and significantly lessen the pain from arthritis. However, one glucosamine product can be very different from another. Glucosamine provided in liquid form is absorbed more quickly, much more fully, and provides greater and longer-lasting relief than glucosamine in pill form. Follow the label dosage instructions.

MSM (organic sulphur)

In recent years, MSM has become one of the best-selling herbal remedies for the treatment of arthritic conditions. This herb, extracted from tree bark, is an organic sulphur that can replace the natural sulphurs that are easily destroyed in the food we eat.

Many companies supply petrochemical MSM. However, try to ensure that your purchase is petrochemical-free. (For details of a supplier of petrochemical-free MSM see the Useful Addresses section.) MSM is available in tablet form, vegetarian capsules or powder to blend with food or drinks. The suggested dosage is one to six grams a day.

Garlic (Allium sativum)

Consuming garlic has long been recommended for the prevention and treatment of gout. It is most effective when taken in aged supplement form, as this enhances the medicinal properties and removes the taste and smell. Follow the label dosage instructions.

Organic cider vinegar

Organic cider vinegar is reputed to help break down the acidic deposits in and around the joints. The suggested medicinal dose is one dessertspoonful in a glass of water with a little honey to taste, three times a day.

Suggested menus

Note that the cup you should use for the measures given below is a small teacup or American cup measure rather than a mug. Any helpings of meat, poultry or fish should be no larger than the palm of your hand. Drinks are not included.

Day 1
Breakfast: 1 grapefruit followed by 2 slices of toast
Snack: $\frac{1}{3}$ cup mixed sunflower seeds and almonds
Lunch: Salad with cottage cheese and chives
Snack: 1 cup cherries (if you are not already eating these every day)

| Dinner: | Irish stew with a very small amount of lean beef |
| Snack: | 2 oatcakes |

Day 2

Breakfast:	Porridge with cracked linseed, honey and rice milk, 1 tofu yoghurt
Snack:	1 banana
Lunch:	2 soft-poached eggs on wholemeal toast, 1 potato scone
Snack:	$\frac{1}{3}$ cup pecan nuts
Dinner:	Grilled chicken breast with potatoes, carrots and parsnips
Snack:	$\frac{1}{3}$ cup dried apricots

Day 3

Breakfast:	1 large wedge of canteloupe melon, 2 Ryvita wafers
Snack:	1 carob bar (available from healthfood shops)
Lunch:	1 large baked potato with tuna, 2 oatcakes
Snack:	$\frac{1}{3}$ cup mixed dried fruit and nuts
Dinner:	Home-made chicken curry with brown rice, pear
Snack:	2 slices wholemeal toast with jam

Day 4

Breakfast:	Muesli with low-fat milk and chopped banana
Snack:	2 oatcakes
Lunch:	Tomato soup with roll, 1 yoghurt
Snack:	$\frac{1}{3}$ cup dried apricots
Dinner:	Grilled wild salmon with potatoes, broccoli and carrots
Snack:	1 cup cherries

Day 5

Breakfast:	Porridge with cracked linseed, honey and soya milk, 2 Ryvita wafers
Snack:	$\frac{1}{3}$ cup pecan nuts
Lunch:	2 grilled kippers with grilled tomatoes and scrambled egg

Snack: 2 kiwi fruit
Dinner: Mixed vegetable casserole, rice pudding made with
            rice milk
Snack: 2 slices wholemeal toast

Day 6
Breakfast: Fresh fruit salad, soft-boiled egg with toast fingers
Snack: 2 oatcakes
Lunch: Baked potato with cottage cheese and pineapple,
            slice of carob cake
Snack: $\frac{1}{3}$ cup mixed nuts
Dinner: Falafel (similar to a veggie burger and available
            from healthfood shops) with chips baked in the
            oven (see p. 40)
Snack: 1 orange

Day 7
Breakfast: 2 slices wholemeal toast with raw honey, banana
Snack: 2 rice cakes (available from healthfood shops)
Lunch: Mixed salad, baked apple
Snack: Pear
Dinner: Baked wild salmon with potatoes, broccoli and
            carrots
Snack: 1 slice carrot cake

5

Complementary Therapies

Complementary medicine has been described as all the therapies
not taught in medical school. It includes such techniques as
acupuncture, homeopathy and reflexology. You may know these
as 'alternative therapies' – but this term can be misleading. The
word alternative suggests that the therapy can be used to replace
conventional medicine. Unfortunately, in treating gout this is
rarely the case.

Complementary therapies are suitable for treating disease for
the following reasons:

- they have non-invasive qualities;
- they are largely free from side effects;
- they can be used in addition to long-term medication;
- most of them are enjoyable.

People who use complementary therapies do report substantial
benefits, although some of these may derive from simply
knowing that they are doing something positive to help themselves. Different therapies appear to suit different people.

Acupressure

Acupressure is an ancient form of oriental healing, combining
acupuncture and massage. Practitioners of this technique use the
thumb, fingertip or the palm of the hand to firmly massage certain
pressure points located at specific sites throughout the body.
These points are the same as those used in acupuncture (see
below). Neither oils nor equipment are used in this type of
therapy.

Acupressure is believed to enhance the body's own healing
mechanisms. Pain relief is sometimes rapid. However, improvements can take longer in chronic conditions. At some hospitals in

the UK, acupressure is available as part of the physiotherapy treatment options.

Acupuncture

Also an ancient form of oriental healing, acupuncture involves puncturing the skin with fine needles at specific points in the body. These points are located along energy channels (meridians) that are believed to correspond to certain internal organs. The energy itself is known as chi. Needles are inserted to increase, decrease or unblock the flow of chi energy so that the balance of yin and yang is restored. Yin, the female force, is calm and passive; it also represents dark, cold, swelling and moisture. On the other hand, yang, the male force, is stimulating and aggressive, representing heat, light, contraction and dryness. It is thought that an imbalance in these forces is the cause of illness and disease. For example, a person who feels the cold, and suffers fluid retention and fatigue, would be considered to have an excess of yin. A person suffering from headaches, however, will be deemed to have an excess of yang.

Emotional, physical or environmental factors are believed to disturb the chi energy balance, and can also be treated. For example, acupuncture has been used to alleviate stress, digestive disorders, insomnia, asthma and allergies. Studies have shown that treatment promotes the brain to release endorphins and encephalins (natural painkillers), boost the immune system and calm the nervous system. It can be seen, then, that acupuncture has many applications.

A qualified acupuncturist will use a set method to determine acupuncture points – it is thought that there are as many as 2,000 such points on the body. At a consultation, questions may be asked about lifestyle, sleeping patterns, fears, phobias and reactions to stress. The pulses will be felt, then the acupuncture itself carried out, fine needles being placed in the relevant sites. The first consultation will normally last an hour, and patients should feel improvements after four to six sessions.

In treating gout, this traditional Chinese medicine advocates that an overrich diet causes a build-up of damp and heat internally, causing phlegm to stagnate and bringing about disturbance of the spleen and kidneys. Treatment, therefore, involves placing fine needles in the spleen and stomach acupuncture points. Other local points are used according to the joint affected by gout.

In one important study in China,[7] 54 sufferers of arthritic disease were given a form of acupuncture (warm needling in this case) in which the needles are dipped in Zhuifengsu, a Chinese herb. As a consequence, every sufferer reported a decrease in their pain. In another study, in Russia, into auriculo-electropuncture (AEP)[8] – treatment of acupuncture points on the ear – all 16 arthritis sufferers felt better after treatment, showing 'statistically significant' improvement in their blood samples. The results of these studies are believed to apply to all types of arthritis, including gout.

Acupuncture is now losing its unorthodox reputation, and has made much headway in the West. In recent years it has gained so much respect in the medical field that many doctors now perform the therapy.

Bioelectromagnetics

Bioelectromagnetics is the study of how living organisms – all of which produce electrical currents – interact with magnetic fields. The electrical currents within our bodies are capable of creating magnetic fields that extend outside our bodies, and these fields can be influenced by external magnetic forces. In fact, specific external magnetism can actually produce physical and behavioural changes. Just as drugs induce a response in their target tissues, so low magnetic fields can produce a chosen biological response – but without the chemical side effects associated with drugs.

External magnetism cannot only correct abnormalities in the energy fields of patients with disease, effectively working as a healer, it is also capable of stabilizing a chronic condition –

although certainly not in every case. As a pain reliever, external magnetism is becoming ever more widely used, and much experimentation is currently under way. Electromagnetic apparatus is even becoming a regular fixture of NHS treatment rooms. This apparatus creates a pulsed magnetic field, which is used to aid the recovery of bone fractures, tendon and ligament tears and muscle injuries, for example. A small, light, comparatively inexpensive version can be purchased for easy-to-wear home use. External magnetism should not be used by anyone fitted with a heart pacemaker.

External magnetism in the form of a specially designed wrist appliance – worn like a wristwatch – is also believed to be effective in treating aches, pains and injuries in any region of the body. As with other types of external magnetism, this appliance is said to improve the ability of the blood to carry oxygen and nutrients around the body. It is also believed to speed the removal of toxins and other waste products. Various appliances are available for use on different parts of the body (see the Useful Addresses section for outlet details).

Homeopathy

The homeopathic approach to medicine is holistic: this means that the overall health of a person, physical, emotional and psychological, is assessed before treatment commences. The homeopathic belief is that the whole make-up of a person determines the disorders to which he or she is prone, and their likely symptoms. After a thorough consultation, the homeopath will offer a remedy compatible with the patient's symptoms as well as with their temperament and characteristics. Consequently, two individuals with the same disorder may be offered entirely different remedies.

Homeopathic remedies are derived from plant, mineral and animal substances, which are soaked in alcohol to extract what are known as the 'live' ingredients. This initial solution is then diluted many times, being vigorously shaken each time to add energy. Impurities are removed and the remaining solution made up into tablets, ointments, powders or suppositories. Interestingly, low dilution remedies are used for severe symptoms while high dilution remedies are used for milder symptoms.

Since antiquity, the homeopathic concept has been that 'like cures like'. The full healing abilities of this type of remedy were first recognized in the early nineteenth century, when a German doctor, Samuel Hahnemann, noticed that the herbal cure for malaria – which was based on an extract of cinchona bark (quinine) – actually produced symptoms of malaria. Further tests convinced him that the production of mild symptoms caused the body to fight the disease. He went on to treat malaria patients successfully with dilute doses of cinchona bark.

Each homeopathic remedy is first 'proved' by being taken by a healthy person – usually a volunteer homeopath – and having the symptoms noted. This remedy is then known to be capable of curing the same symptoms in an ill person. The whole idea of proving and using homeopathic remedies can be difficult to comprehend as it is exactly the opposite to how conventional medicines operate. For example, a patient who has a cold with a runny nose would be treated with a homeopathic remedy that would produce a runny nose in a healthy patient. Conventional medicine, on the other hand, would provide something that blocks up the nose.

Nowadays, a homeopathic remedy can be formulated to aid virtually every disorder. Although remedies are safe and non-addictive, occasionally the patient's symptoms may briefly worsen. This is known as a healing crisis and is usually short-lived. It is actually a good indication that the remedy is working well.

You should visit a homeopath if you have a medical problem that is not getting better or if you are continually swapping one set of symptoms for another. It is a common misconception that you can just pop along to your local chemist, look up your particular complaint on the homeopathic remedy chart and begin taking the remedy. If only it were that simple: homeopathic training takes several years, and a lot of knowledge and experience is required before practitioners can decide the correct remedies for complaints other than the very superficial. And as I mentioned earlier, what works for one person is not liable to work for another.

Selecting an appropriate remedy is only part of the procedure, however. The homeopath will also evaluate patient reaction to ascertain what, if any, further treatment is necessary.

Hydrotherapy (1)

In 400 BC, Hippocrates alleged that bathing was useful for a variety of conditions, and he included gout in his list. A long soak in a hot bath is profoundly relaxing. It also has a calming effect on the central nervous system. Even more soothing, surprisingly, is a long soak in a bath as close as possible to body temperature (37°C). For best results, the bathwater should cover your shoulders – and the longer you are immersed, the better you will feel. For comfort, place a folded towel beneath your head – although the water should provide adequate support as a body in water weighs only a quarter of its normal weight. Keep the temperature of the water as constant as possible by regularly topping up from the hot tap.

You may be interested to know that heart size increases by 30 per cent within six seconds of immersion in warm water, cardiac output increases by 34 per cent, blood pressure remains steady and changes within the sympathetic nervous system mean that there is a decreased perception of pain.

Hydrotherapy (2)

It is important for a person with gout to drink plenty of fluids. This reduces the risk of uric acid crystallizing in the joints (the cause of the severe pain in acute gout). Ideally, you should try to drink as much as 3.5 litres (6 pints) of water a day. It is fine to include other fluids in this amount, such as fruit juices and herbal teas. Try topping up fruit juices with water and keep a glass at your work station or in the kitchen so you can keep taking sips. If you can't manage to drink the recommended amount, don't worry – just drink as much as you can.

Hypnotherapy

Hypnotherapy may be described as psychotherapy using hypnosis. There is, however, still no acceptable definition for the actual state of hypnosis. It is commonly described as an altered state of consciousness, lying somewhere between being awake and asleep. People under hypnosis are aware of their surroundings, yet their minds are, to a large extent, under the control of the hypnotist. People under hypnosis also seem to pass control of their actions, as well as a chunk of their thoughts, to the hypnotist. We have all seen people under hypnosis on TV, acting out a role. At the time they are absorbed in what they have been told to do – often instigated by a specific trigger word – but immediately afterwards they wonder what on earth they were doing. Their behaviour had been dictated, to a certain degree, by the hypnotist. Hypnotherapy is about the hypnotist using this power for therapeutic purposes, and it is performed by the therapist putting the patient into a trance.

By the early nineteenth century, some physicians were using hypnotism – then called mesmerism – to perform pain-free operations. The majority of medical professionals were highly sceptical, however, believing that the patients had been either schooled – or paid – to show no pain. Not until the last two decades has hypnotism become an accepted form of therapy.

Nowadays, a hypnotherapist will take a full psychological and physiological history of each patient, and then will slowly talk the patient into a trance state. The therapist can either use direct suggestion – by indicating that the patient's pain, for example, will notably lessen – or will begin to explore the root cause of any tension, anxiety or depression.

Hypnotherapists have found that when, in chronic pain conditions, the level of tension is lowered, many of the physical symptoms are also greatly reduced. Some experts in the field believe that the main purpose of hypnotherapy is to aid relaxation, reduce tension and increase confidence and the ability to cope with problems. However, there has been at least one study into the effects of hypnotherapy on arthritic conditions. In this instance,[9] levels of beta endorphin, epinephrine, norepine-phrine, dopamine and serotonin were measured in 19 patients before and after hypnosis. Following the therapy there were clinically and statistically significant decreases in pain, anxiety and depression, and increases in the endorphins that have a beneficial effect on the immune system. The conclusion was that hypnotherapy could well play an important role in conquering arthritic conditions, including gout.

One common fear is that the therapist may, while the patient is in a trance, implant dangerous suggestions or extract improper personal information. I can only say that patients can come out of a trance at any time – particularly if they are asked to do or say anything they would not even contemplate when awake. And malpractice would only have to be brought to light once to ruin the therapist's career. You may prefer to visit a hypnotherapist recommended by your doctor.

Relaxation and meditation

You may wonder how relaxation techniques and meditation can help a person with gout. Well, any activity that increases energy demands also increases the metabolism, which then produces uric acid. Stress increases the metabolism and is a common trigger of gout attacks. Avoiding stress is therefore important in gout.

Deep-breathing exercises are an important prelude to relaxation, excellent for achieving and maintaining overall health, and can be invaluable in reducing the intense pain of a flare-up of gout. Meditation has been shown in research to help normalize blood pressure and boost the immune system, both of which are of great benefit to people with gout.

Deep breathing

In normal breathing, we take oxygen from the atmosphere down into our lungs. The diaphragm contracts, and air is pulled into the chest cavity. When we breathe out, we expel carbon dioxide and other waste gases back into the atmosphere. But when we are stressed or upset, we tend to use the rib muscles to expand the chest. We breathe more quickly, sucking in shallowly. This is good in a crisis as it allows us to obtain the optimum amount of oxygen in the shortest possible time, providing our bodies with the extra power needed to handle the emergency.

Some people do tend to get stuck in chest-breathing mode. Long-term shallow breathing is not only detrimental to our physical and emotional health, it can also lead to hyperventilation, panic attacks, chest pains, dizziness and gastro-intestinal problems.

To test your breathing, ask yourself:

- How fast are you breathing as you are reading this?
- Are you pausing between breaths?
- Are you breathing with your chest or with your diaphragm?

A *breathing exercise*

The following deep-breathing exercise should, ideally, be performed daily:

1 Make yourself comfortable, either sitting or lying, in a warm room where you know you will be alone for at least half an hour.
2 Close your eyes and try to relax.
3 Gradually slow down your breathing, inhaling and exhaling as evenly as possible.
4 Place one hand on your chest and the other on your abdomen, just below your ribcage.
5 As you inhale, allow your abdomen to swell outwards (your chest should barely move).
6 As you exhale, let your abdomen flatten.

Give yourself a few minutes to get into a smooth, easy rhythm. As worries and distractions arise, don't hang on to them. Wait calmly for them to float out of your mind – then focus once more on your breathing.

When you feel ready to end the exercise, open your eyes. Allow yourself time to become alert before rolling on to one side and getting up. With practice, you will begin breathing with your diaphragm quite naturally – and in times of stress you should be able to correct your breathing without too much effort.

A relaxation exercise

Relaxation is one of the forgotten skills in today's hectic world. We already know that stress – which can give rise to muscle tension, insomnia, hypertension and depression – is one of the greatest enemies of the gout sufferer. It is advisable, therefore, to learn at least one relaxation technique.

The following exercise is perhaps the easiest:

1 Make yourself comfortable in a place where you will not be disturbed – listening to restful music may help you relax.
2 Begin to slow down your breathing, inhaling through your nose to a count of one, two – ensuring that the abdomen pushes outwards, as explained.
3 Exhale to a count of one, two, three, four – or up to five and six.
4 After a couple of minutes, concentrate on each part of the body in turn, starting with your right arm. Consciously relax each set of muscles, allowing the tension to flow right out. Let your arm feel heavier and heavier as every last remnant of tension seeps away. Follow this procedure with the muscles of your left arm, then the muscles of your face, your neck, your stomach, your hips and finally your legs.

Visualization

When you have achieved step four of the relaxation exercise, a technique called visualization can be introduced. As you continue to breathe slowly and evenly, imagine yourself surrounded, perhaps, by lush, peaceful countryside, beside a gently trickling stream – or maybe on a deserted tropical beach, beneath swaying palm fronds, listening to the sounds of the ocean, thousands of miles from your worries and cares. Let the warm sun, the gentle breeze, the peacefulness of it all wash over you.

The tranquillity you feel at this stage can be enhanced by frequently repeating the exercise – once or twice a day is best.

With time, you should be able to switch into a calm state of mind whenever you feel stressed.

Meditation

Arguably the oldest natural therapy, meditation is the simplest and most effective form of self-help. Dr Herbert Benson of the Harvard Medical School has been able to show that meditation tends to normalize blood pressure, the pulse rate and the level of stress hormones in the blood. He has also proved that it produces changes in brainwave patterns, which show less excitability, and that it improves the white blood cell (immune) response as well as hormone response. It must therefore be considered an important and easily accessible aid to recovery for people who suffer from gout.

The unusual thing about meditation is that it involves letting go, allowing the mind to roam freely. However, as most of us are used to endeavouring to control our thoughts – in our work, for example – letting go is not as easy as it sounds.

It may help to know that people who regularly meditate say they have more energy, require less sleep, are less anxious and feel far more alive than before they did so. Ideally, the technique should be taught by a teacher – but as meditation is essentially performed alone, it can be learnt alone with equal success.

Meditation may, to some people, sound a bit offbeat. But isn't it worth a try – especially when you can do it for free? Kick off those shoes and make yourself comfortable, somewhere you can be alone for a while. Now follow these simple instructions:

1 Close your eyes, relax, and practise the deep-breathing exercise as described.
2 Concentrate on your breathing. Try to free your mind of conscious control. Letting it roam unchecked, try to allow the deeper, more serene part of you to take over.
3 If you wish to go further into meditation, concentrate now on mentally repeating a mantra – a certain word or phrase. It should be something positive, such as 'relax', 'I feel calm', 'I am feeling much better' or even 'I am special'.

4 When you are ready to finish, open your eyes and allow yourself time to adjust to the outside world before getting to your feet.

The aim of mentally repeating a mantra is to plant the positive thought into your subconscious mind. It is a form of self-hypnosis, but you alone control the messages placed in your mind.

Mineral tissue salts

Mineral tissue salts therapy is an offshoot of homeopathy and thus completely safe. As with most complementary therapies, this one can be used in conjunction with conventional medication without any side effects. Mineral tissue salts are reputed to be of particular benefit where the body is overly acidic, as is the case for people with gout. They are also useful for treating minor illnesses, from skin conditions to sinus disorders.

The original 12 remedies were isolated by Dr Wilhelm Schuessler in 1880. The natural ingredients are homeopathically prepared to a potency that is reputed to allow the cells to rebalance their salts content, to restore health. The tiny white tablets dissolve in the mouth, leaving a pleasant taste. There are more than 30 different tissue salts in all, but the most useful for gout patients are No. 10 Nat. Phos (sodium phosphate) and, for use during an attack of gout on account of its inflammatory properties, No. 4 Ferr. Phos (iron phosphate). Before you start a course of tissue salts, make sure you read the label instructions.

Mineral tissue salts are available from healthfood shops and chemists.

Reflexology

Reflexology, an ancient oriental therapy, has only recently been adopted in the West. It operates on the proposition that the body is divided into different energy zones, all of which can be exploited in the prevention and treatment of any disorder.

Reflexologists have identified ten energy channels, beginning in the toes and extending to the fingers and the top of the head. Each channel relates to a particular bodily zone and to the organs in that zone. For example, the big toe relates to the head – the brain, sinus area, neck, pituitary glands, eyes and ears. By applying pressure to the appropriate terminal in the form of a small, specialized massage, a practitioner can determine which energy pathways are blocked.

Experts in this type of manipulative therapy claim that all the organs of the body are reflected in the feet. They also believe that reflexology aids the removal of waste products and blockages within the energy channels, improving circulation and gland function. Reflexology is certainly relaxing. Indeed, many patients fall asleep during the therapy. Because my own feet are so ticklish, I felt I had cause to worry before my first reflexology session (I could imagine myself involuntarily kicking the therapist). Fortunately, I quickly found that the sensations were pleasurable and I was able to relax – and I must say I was surprised to note how accurate the therapist was in detecting my own indispositions.

Therapists certainly do exert pressure on the tiny crystalline deposits of uric acid that we all have on our feet. However, the idea that the deposits are broken up by reflexology and absorbed into the body's waste disposal system is a matter for debate. The crystals of uric acid present in gout are manifestations of a physical problem experienced by the body rather than within the energy field.

Many therapists prefer to take down a full case history before commencing treatment. Each session will take up to 45 minutes (the preliminary session will take longer), and you will be treated either sitting in a chair or lying down, depending on the therapist and on the patient's condition. There is much ongoing research into the effectiveness of reflexology on arthritic conditions. In fact, it has been known for patients to reduce the intake of cortisone drugs – with their physician's consent, of course – following a course of reflexology treatment.

6
Emotional Help

Gout can affect every area of your life. In the early stages of the illness, sufferers are often beset by fears for the future, concerns about the effectiveness of the medications they are prescribed and anxieties about their ability to alter their diet and lifestyle. They are likely even to feel anger over the way gout is viewed by the general public – or even worse, by their families and friends. These factors can be major sources of upset. However, given time, education and self-awareness training, gout sufferers can gradually come to terms with the condition, finding ways to cope effectively with the stress, the reactions of others and any further outbreaks of pain.

A chronic illness

Even when people with gout are doing all within their power to control the condition – and doing it with success – they will always be predisposed to developing it again. Once gout has reared its ugly head, it sits in the shadows, just waiting to leap out should you put a foot wrong. For this reason, gout is considered a chronic condition, just like all arthritic disease.

It's an unfortunate fact that chronic illness creates a plethora of negative emotions. These emotions are discussed below.

I feel so angry!
When you learn that the searing pain is likely to return, that you must now make permanent and drastic changes to your life, you may feel very angry. After all, your friends are able to continue to enjoy a few beers at the pub, they can eat as much meat as they like, and they haven't been told to lose weight – forgive me if these are not your particular problems, but I'm sure you see what I mean. If it is kidney disease that has brought about your gout, or even medications for another health problem, then that could

easily be another cause of anger. After all, you are suffering from one disorder already – it doesn't seem fair that it should have led to another.

It may help to know that anger is a natural response to the diagnosis of chronic disease, and that it is generally followed by acceptance – albeit grudging. I'm afraid the only way to get on top of this illness is to take positive action. It distracts attention from any negative emotions and gives a clear focus.

I feel so afraid!

Of course you feel afraid when you develop an illness for which there is, as yet, no safe and absolute cure. Fears tend to centre around the future, and what will become of you. You may be afraid of repeated attacks; afraid that they will be more painful each time; afraid of the long-term effects of medication; afraid to tell people of the nature of your illness; afraid of being laughed at; afraid of being unable to make the necessary changes to your diet and lifestyle – the list goes on.

There is no doubt that chronic illness exerts a profound effect on the individual. However, most people with gout will say that the fear of the unknown abates with time. Sufferers learn that they can still take great pleasure from family life, enjoy social occasions, take up interests and hobbies and be of use to others. Most importantly, people with gout learn that their condition really can be controlled with a little self-determination and the support of their family and friends.

I feel so confused!

After a diagnosis of gout it is common to feel confused. Your doctor may have mentioned medications, but you may be baffled about which you should take, and about their long-term effects. You are likely even to be confused about what steps you need to take to help normalize your hyperuricemia. There is so much to absorb in the early days, especially if you are keen to do what you can to help yourself. You may rest assured, however, that your doctor will know which medications are most suited to your particular needs, and that he or she will be able to guide you through any diet and lifestyle changes you wish to try. It's always helpful to gather together as much information as possible about your condition – from your doctor, pharmacist, bookshop, library and the Internet. It will all help clarify matters. Then take it one step at a time.

I feel so vulnerable!

Vulnerability is a natural human condition. We all need people to love us; we all crave the affirmation of others. To a large extent we are all dependent upon others, measuring their responses in order to reassure ourselves that we are worthwhile human beings, that we are indeed loveable. When an individual has an illness that is perceived as unglamorous and brought about by overindulgence, it can be easy to feel unattractive, unappealing. It is even possible to feel no longer loveable.

Feelings of vulnerability will always be present in chronic illness, but to a large extent they can be defeated by looking less to outsiders for affirmation. We all have inner strengths and particular talents, even some of which we may at first be unaware. Yet if we waited for others to point them out we would probably be waiting for ever! Your particular forte may lie in planning and organizing, or problem solving or handling finances – not necessarily out of the family setting. You may be an authority on steam engines, a good listener, a talented artist, an excellent singer, a diligent student, a competent driver – the possibilities are endless. Do not underestimate yourself!

Remember, too, that the people who love you will not stop doing so because you suffer from gout. Love is about who you are – your character and personality, your strengths and weaknesses – your *inner* self. A disease with an unglamorous reputation isn't going to change things.

I feel so guilty!

Feelings of guilt are common in chronic illness. It is natural to want to lay the blame for falling ill at someone's door, and many sufferers imagine they themselves must have done something wrong to deserve such retribution. But blaming either yourself or others is pointless. Life is a lottery. Some people are rich, some poor; some clever, some not so clever; some fall ill, some remain healthy. That's just the way it is.

You may, after learning that improvement lies mainly in your hands, feel guilty about making no real progress. But assuming you have tried to help yourself, there is probably a sound reason for your failure. For example, you may be held back by additional health problems, or you may not have allowed sufficient time for any improvements to show.

I can't accept that I have a chronic disease!

Refusal to accept the needs of the condition is unfortunately very common – but again, it is a very natural response. After a first flare-up and a diagnosis of gout, it can be easy to believe that there will be no recurrence, that it will all go away. I have even come across people who have suffered several attacks and still blithely believe that each is the last. Unfortunately, attacks of gout will always recur if nothing is done to improve the situation. Not only that, the attacks will become increasingly painful and likely to spread to further areas. The knock-on effects of untreated gout attacks can be kidney disease, high blood pressure and heart disease, as already explained.

In my research, it has also become clear that a number of gout sufferers refuse to make the necessary changes to their diet and lifestyle. They have eaten meat and drunk beer all their lives and have no intention of changing now. It's as if they have an impenetrable field around them that will protect them from future health risks. I'm afraid it doesn't quite work that way.

Dealing with other people

The reactions of others can be one of the most difficult aspects of gout. As I noted at the beginning of this book, in the past the condition was ridiculed mercilessly and the general public was left in no doubt that overindulgence was the cause. So how do you cope when the people around you poke fun at you, when they only laugh and tell you you've brought it on yourself? Read on and you will hopefully find some answers.

How can I make people take my condition seriously?

Without doubt, some people are incredibly insensitive. You may feel that you are always on your guard, dreading the remark that will send you into a whirl of anger or the depths of despair. Sadly, developing a condition like gout lays you open to the preconceptions of others. You really should not have to grin and bear the sniggers, the hurtful remarks. Instead, it would be best to try to tell the person, very calmly, that gout is exceedingly painful and no laughing matter.

Standing up for yourself is not easy, but doing so can have a releasing effect – unlike when you fake indifference or clam up and walk away. In such instances, you may end up feeling hurt, offended and very resentful. Your most intense feeling, however, will probably be anger – at the other person and at yourself, for allowing yourself to be hurt.

Dealing with others

It is generally when a person first announces that they have gout that they face the worst of the hurtful remarks. To counter that, it is probably best to arm yourself with as much information on the subject as possible, so that you can show them that gout is a serious matter. If the joking continues, it is important for your self-esteem that you tackle those responsible more firmly. For instance, if someone close to you says, 'You must really be living it up – no wonder you've got gout!' you could reply something like, 'Actually, I'm trying very hard to follow the recommended diet – but it isn't easy.' They may reply jokingly that you can't be trying very hard, to which you might reply, 'I'm trying as hard as I can. As a matter of fact I would appreciate some support from you in this – gout isn't an easy condition to conquer.' They will probably really start to listen at this point, which gives you the chance to explain any difficulties you're having.

A condition like gout is much easier to handle when you have the support of your family and friends. However, there may always be some people who fail to see past the old stigma and continue to chuckle at the mention of the word gout. In cases like this, it is best to try to harden your heart to those people. It is their misfortune to possess an inflexible mind – and to have lost your respect.

Self-talk

The way we speak to ourselves has great bearing on our stress levels – and as already stated, stress is a common trigger of attacks of gout. When we analyse our thoughts, we are often surprised at their negativity – but they must be examined before we can begin to change their destructive pattern. When the TV breaks down, for example, your initial thoughts may be, 'It's so unfair! I was really looking forward to watching that film!' 'This is all I need! I can't afford a new set!' 'If the set can be repaired, it will probably cost a small fortune!' 'What am I supposed to do with my time – sit twiddling my thumbs?' Stress-provoking thoughts by any standard!

By being aware that negative thoughts create stress, you can train yourself into more positive self-talk. Using the same example, you may, instead, think: 'I'll ring around for quotes in the morning – maybe it won't cost much to repair.' 'It was on its last legs anyway – I'll take the opportunity to buy a more up-to-date set.' 'I could buy a new set using hire purchase.' 'I could buy a reconditioned set if I can't afford a new one.' 'I could rent one and not have to worry about repair costs.' 'In the meantime, this is my chance to read that book, to finish my tapestry, to phone Aunt Betty.'

The following examples of stress-relieving self-talk can be applied to many potentially stressful situations:

'I'll break this problem into separate sections – they'll be easier to handle.'
'I'll take things one step at a time.'
'Is this really worth getting upset and angry over?'
'I've coped before, so I'll cope again.'
'I can always ask for help if I need it.'
'It could have been much worse.'

'This is hardly a matter of life or death!'
'There's nothing I can do about this situation, so I'll have to
accept it.'

Lifestyle measures to help prevent gout

Here, in brief, is a reminder of the lifestyle measures necessary
for lowering uric acid levels and correcting hyperuricemia:

- Cut down on foods containing purines – meat, poultry and fish
  (particularly organ meat and shellfish), gravies, asparagus,
  cauliflower and so on.
- Beware of different eating and drinking patterns, for example
  on holiday. Before travelling, ask your doctor to prescribe a
  medication that can be taken at the first sign of gout. In most
  cases, this will stop the episode in its tracks.
- Try to eat half a dozen cherries every day.
- Take the recommended supplements.
- Maintain a healthy weight – avoid crash dieting.
- Drink plenty of water.
- Cut down on your alcohol consumption.
- Avoid joint injury, if at all possible.
- Avoid stress.

Action for acute attacks

Flare-ups of pain are an ever-present risk in gout. They can be
caused by:

- injury to an area affected by gout in the past – a stubbed toe,
  for example;
- a sharp increase in alcohol consumption;
- surgery;
- illness;
- an infection;
- eating more purine foods than normal;

- not eating enough food (starvation);
- not drinking enough water;
- use of certain prescription drugs.

The following pointers should help you to cope with an attack:

1 Take action as soon as you recognize that an attack is occurring. This may include immediate rest, alternate heat and cold application, painkilling medication – even sending someone out to the shop to buy you some cherries. Remember that you should eat or drink no high-purine foods once an attack is under way. A therapeutic diet – for the duration of the attack – should come largely from cheese, milk, eggs and low-purine vegetables.

2 Be positive! A positive frame of mind can speed recovery. Tell yourself, 'I'll get through this just as I have before.' 'I am more aware of how to help myself this time.' 'I'll make efforts to distract myself from the pain.' 'I won't let myself get depressed – that will do me more harm than good.'

3 Explore the possible reasons for the increase in pain. Ask yourself, 'Did I eat too much food that contains purines; did I drink too much alcohol?' Maybe in an effort to lose weight you have not been eating enough?

4 Decide how you can reduce the risk of future flare-ups. If you know where you went wrong, take steps to avoid doing so in future.

5 Review the effectiveness of your current flare-up strategy. Are your present medications adequate in a crisis? Is it time to visit your doctor again? Can you do anything further to stay positive? Could you try a new type of complementary therapy?

Useful Addresses

Arthritis Care
18 Stephenson Way
London NW1 2HD
Tel: 020 7380 6500
Fax: 020 7380 6505
Helpline: 080 8800 4050 (12–4pm weekdays only)
Website: www.arthritiscare.org.uk

For information and advice on all aspects of arthritis. There are over 500 local branches, and Young Arthritis Care (for anybody with arthritis who is under 45) has its own groups, local contacts, and magazines.

Arthritis Foundation
PO Box 7669
Atlanta
GA 30357-0669
USA
Tel: 00 1 800 283 7800
Website: www.arthritis.org.uk

The Arthritis Research Campaign (ARC)
Copeman House
St Mary's Court
St Mary's Gate
Chesterfield
Derbyshire S41 7TD
Tel: 0870 850 5000

Association of Reflexologists
27 Old Gloucester Street
London WC1N 3XX
Tel: 0870 567 3320
Website: www.aor.org.uk
Email: info@aor.org.uk

British Acupuncture Council
63 Jeddo Road
London W12 9HQ
Tel: 020 8735 0400
Website: www.acupuncture.org.uk
Email: info@acupuncture.org.uk

British Homeopathic Association
Hahnemann House
29 Park Street West
Luton LU1 3BE
Tel: 0870 444 3950
Fax: 0870 444 3960
Website: www.trusthomeopathy.org.uk

British Nutrition Foundation
High Holborn House
52–54 High Holborn
London WC1V 6RQ
Tel: 020 7404 6504
Fax: 020 7404 6747
Website: www.nutrition.org.uk
Email: postbox@nutrition.org.uk

Norso Biomagnetics
15 Cotswold View
The Hollow
Bath BA2 1HA
Tel: 01225 314096
Fax: 01225 316397
Website: www.norso–biomagnetics.co.uk
Email: norsouk@aol.com

The Nutri Centre
Lower Ground Floor
The Hale Clinic
7 Park Crescent
London W1B 1PF

Tel: 020 7436 5122 (orders for supplements)
Fax: 020 7436 5171
Website: www.nutricentre.com
Email: enq@nutricentre.com

For good quality supplements and subscription to the regular *Nutri News* publication.

The Nutrition-Mission
6 Havelocks
Crook Farm
Glen Road
Baildon
Shipley
West Yorkshire BD17 5ED
Tel: 01274 590383 or 07970 059493
Website: www.nutrition-mission.co.uk
Email: steve@nutrition-mission.co.uk

Supplies an excellent one-a-day high antioxidant containing over 30 ingredients including the B vitamins and high-dose pantothenic acid and omega 3 and omega 6 essential fatty acids (which are highly recommended in gout). Also supplies Liver Support (which gets the liver and gall bladder working properly) and Intestinal Tone (which balances the gut flora and removes toxins from the body, helping to ease constipation or diarrhoea, flatulence and bloating).

Society of Homeopaths
11 Brookfield
Duncan Close
Moulton Park
Northampton NN3 6WL
Tel: 0845 450 6611
Website: www.homeopathy–soh.org
Email: info@homeopathy–soh.org

Weight Watchers (UK)
3rd Floor North Wing
Hines Meadow
St Cloud Way
Maidenhead
Berkshire SL6 8XB
Website: www.weightwatchers.co.uk

For details on Weight Watchers meetings in the UK, write to:
Weight Watchers (UK) Ltd
Millennium House
Ludlow Road
Maidenhead
Berkshire SL6 2SL

For details on Weight Watchers meetings in Northern Ireland, write to:
Weight Watchers Ireland
1 Phibsboro Road
Dublin 7

References

1 P. Thiehle and H.E. Schroder, 'Epidemiology and pathogenesis of disorders of purine metabolism', *Ter Arkh*, 1997, 59 (4), pp. 14–18.

2 H.R. Schumacher Jr, J.A. Boice, D.I. Daikj et al., 'Randomized double-blind trial of etoricoxib and indometacin in the treatment of acute gouty arthritis', *BMJ* 2, 2002: 324: 1488–92.

3 'Cherry diet control for gout and arthritis', *Texas Reports on Biology and Medicine* V8, fall 1950.

4 *The McDougall Program: twelve days to dynamic health*, NAL Books, 1990, p. 312.

5 Wayne State University College of Medicine – reported in *Better Nutrition*, March 1990, v. 52, n. 3, p. 9.

6 C.L. Curtis, S.G. Rees, C.B. Little et al., 'Pathologic indicators of degradation and inflammation in human osteoarthritic cartilage are abrogated by exposure to n-3 fatty acids', *Arthritis and Rheumatism*, 2002, 46, pp. 1544–53.

7 X. Liu, L. Sun, J. Xiao, S. Yin, C. Liu, Q. Li, H. Li and B. Jin, 'Effect of acupuncture and point-injection treatment on immunologic function in rheumatoid arthritis', General Hospital of PLA, Beijing, *Journal of Traditional Chinese Medicine*, September 1993, 13 (3), pp. 174–8.

8 I.N. Ruchkin and A.P. Burdeinyl, 'Auriculo-electropuncture in rheumatoid arthritis (a double-blind study)', *Ter Arkh*, 1987, 59 (12), pp. 26–30.

9 B.B. Domangue, C.G. Margolis, D. Lieberman and H. Kaji, 'Biochemical correlates of hypnoanalgesia in arthritic pain patients', *Journal of Clinical Psychiatry*, June 1985, 46 (6), pp. 235–8.

Further Reading

Bryan Emmerson, *Getting Rid of Gout*, Oxford University Press, 2003.

Rodney Grahame et al., *Gout – The 'At Your Fingertips Guide'*, Class Publishing, 2003.

Margaret Hills, *Curing Arthritis Diet Book*, Sheldon Press, 1989.

Margaret Hills, *Curing Arthritis – The Drug-Free Way*, Sheldon Press, 2004.

Patrick Holford, *The Optimum Nutrition Bible*, Piatkus, 1998.

Leslie Kenton, *The Raw Energy Bible*, Vermilion, 2001.

Linda Lazarides, *Gourmet Nutritional Therapy Cookbook*, Waterfall 2000, 2000.

Lorna Sass, *New Soy Cookbook: Tempting Recipes for Soybeans, Soy Milk, Tofu, Tempeh, Miso and Soy Sauce*, Chronicle Books, 1998.

Index